This breakthrough giy
evaluate your ris.
individualized plan fe

- How to get past the fear of cancer and fight back
- What cholesterol test results mean
- How active women cut their risk of stroke
- Why your heart attack symptoms may be quite different from a man's
- Ten steps to quitting smoking
- Why women over 55 need exercise as much or more than younger women
- What to do if your family medical tree turns up a potentially dangerous trend
- How to create a personal eating plan to beat the odds of the ten top killers in women
- The common screening tests for osteoporosis, what they are, what they cost
- The latest information on Hormone Replacement Therapy—and how to determine if it's right for you
- and much more!

CHARLOTTE LIBOV is the award-winning co-author of *50 Essential Things to Do When the Doctor Says It's Heart Disease* and *The Woman's Heart Book*. She lectures on women's health issues, frequently appears on radio and television, and her articles have appeared in the *New York Times*. Ms. Libov has an M.S. in mental health counseling from the University of Oregon and lives in Bethlehem, Connecticut.

LILA A. WALLIS, M.D., M.A.C.P., is Clinical Professor of Medicine, Cornell University Medical College, Founding President of the National Council on Women's Health, Master of the American College of Physicians, and author of *The Whole Woman Takes Charge of Her Health* (with Marian Betancourt) and *Textbook of Women's Health*.

ALSO BY CHARLOTTE LIBOV

The Woman's Heart Book (with Fredric J. Pashkow, M.D.)
50 Essential Things to Do When the Doctor Says It's Heart Disease
(with Fredric J. Pashkow, M.D.)
Migraine: 50 Essential Things to Do

BEAT YOUR RISK FACTORS

A Woman's Guide to Reducing
Her Risk for Cancer, Heart
Disease, Stroke, Diabetes,
and Osteoporosis

CHARLOTTE LIBOV

Foreword by Lila A. Wallis, M.D.

Ⓟ

A PLUME BOOK

Publisher's Note
The ideas, procedures, and suggestions contained in this book are not intended as a substitute for consulting with your physician. All matters regarding your health require
medical supervision.

PLUME
Published by the Penguin Group
Penguin Putnam Inc., 375 Hudson Street, New York, New York 10014, U.S.A.
Penguin Books Ltd, 27 Wrights Lane, London W8 5TZ, England
Penguin Books Australia Ltd, Ringwood, Victoria, Australia
Penguin Books Canada Ltd, 10 Alcorn Avenue, Toronto, Ontario, Canada M4V 3B2
Penguin Books (N.Z.) Ltd, 182–190 Wairau Road, Auckland 10, New Zealand

Penguin Books Ltd, Registered Offices: Harmondsworth, Middlesex, England

First published by Plume, a member of Penguin Putnam Inc.

First Plume Printing, July, 1999
10 9 8 7 6 5 4 3 2 1

REGISTERED TRADEMARK—MARCA REGISTRADA

Library of Congress Cataloging-in-Publication Data
Libov, Charlotte.
    Beat your risk factors : a woman's guide to reducing her risk for
cancer, heart disease, stroke, diabetes, and osteoporosis /
Charlotte Libov : foreword by Lila A. Wallis.
        p.   cm.
    Includes bibliographical references and index.
    ISBN 0-452-27832-5
    1. Women—Diseases—Risk factors.   2. Women—Diseases—Prevention.
I. Title.
RA778.L7848   1999
616'.0082—DC21   99-22860
                                                            CIP
                                                            Rev.

Printed in the United States of America
Set in Goudy and Copperplate
Designed by Eve L. Kirch

BOOKS ARE AVAILABLE AT QUANTITY DISCOUNTS WHEN USED TO PROMOTE PRODUCTS OR
SERVICES. FOR INFORMATION PLEASE WRITE TO PREMIUM MARKETING DIVISION, PENGUIN PUT-
NAM INC., 375 HUDSON STREET, NEW YORK, NY 10014.

For Terry

CONTENTS

PART THREE: FOUR STEPS TO REDUCING YOUR RISKS

ACKNOWLEDGMENTS

First, I owe a tremendous debt to the following medical experts who willingly shared their expertise with me. They graciously submitted to lengthy interviews and innumerable follow-up questions, and many even reviewed chapter drafts. They include:

Fredric J. Pashkow, M.D., and Douglas Rogers, M.D., the Cleveland Clinic Foundation; Graham Colditz, M.D., and JoAnn Manson, M.D., Harvard Medical School; Patrick Borgen, M.D., John P. Curtin, M.D., Kenneth Offit, M.D., Larry Norton, M.D., Diane Stover, M.D., and Sidney J. Winawer, M.D., Memorial Sloan-Kettering Cancer Center; Curtis Mettlin, Ph.D., and M. Steven Piver, M.D., Rosewell Park Medical Institute; Peter Deckers, M.D., Allen Glassman, M.D., Bernard Greenberg, M.D., Robert Greenstein, M.D., Sharon Kilbride, R.N., B.S.N., O.C.N., Robert Pilarski, M.S., and Jonathan R. Sporn, M.D., University of Connecticut School of Medicine; John Bond, M.D., and Jack Mandel, Ph.D., University of Minnesota; Carol Lee, M.D., Lawrence Brass, M.D., Karl Insogna, M.D., and David Leffell, M.D., who also gave me permission to use some of his material in the skin cancer questionnaire and William S. Beckett, M.D., M.P.H., University of Rochester School of Medicine and Dentistry.

x   ACKNOWLEDGMENTS

Also Barrie Anderson, M.D., University of Iowa Hospital & Clinics; Louis Caplan, M.D., Tufts University School of Medicine; Samuel S. Epstein M.D., University of Illinois School of Public Health; Linda Hershey, M.D., State University of New York at Buffalo; Scott Kuwada, M.D., University of Utah; Susan M. Love, M.D., University of California, Los Angeles; Janet Rose Osuch, M.D., Michigan State University; Cynthia S. Pomerleau, Ph.D., University of Michigan; Joel Posner, M.D., Medical College of Pennsylvania; Gerald Reaven, M.D., Stanford University School of Medicine; Dorothy L. Rosenthal, M.D., Johns Hopkins University; Lila A. Wallis, M.D., Cornell University Medical College; Kathleen Wishner, M.D., University of Southern California; and Jacqueline L. Wolf, M.D., Brigham and Women's Hospital.

Also Lois Jovanovic, M.D., Patricia Hollander, M.D., International Diabetes Center, Minneapolis; Samsun Medical Research Foundation, Santa Barbara, California; Patricia T. Kelly, Ph.D., Salick Health Care Inc., Oakland, California; Joy Kistler, M.S.C.D.E., Joslin Diabetes Center, Boston; Barnett Kramer, M.D., National Institutes of Health; Lamar S. McGinnis, American Cancer Society; and Tom Sheldon, M.D., Nashua Regional Cancer Center, Nashua, New Hampshire.

In addition, Richard Bernstein, M.D., Mamaroneck, New York; Nancy Clark, M.S., R.D., Brookline, Massachusetts; Patricia Davidson, M.D., Washington, D.C.; Sue Gebo, M.P.H., R.D., West Hartford, Connecticut; Saul S. Gusberg, M.D., Dobbs Ferry, New York; Diane Krieger, M.D., Miami, Florida; and Morris Notelovitz, M.D., Ph.D., Gainesville, Florida.

This is a book that took me four years to write, and most of that time was spent conducting interviews with some of the top medical experts in their field. My only fear is that I may have inadvertently omitted someone; if that is the case, my most sincere apologies.

I offer my personal thanks to Jack and Harleen Epstein, Ginnie Lupi, and Ceil Sinnex for their contributions.

Carole Able is not only my literary agent but, I am proud to say, a dear friend. This is the third project I've worked on with my editor, Deborah Brody, and, as usual, I am grateful for her excellent recommendations and her extreme patience.

For her inspiration, Barbara Seaman receives my gratitude. A true pathfinder in the cause of women's health, Barbara was also always ready with encouragement and help.

Rita E. Watson not only co-authored all of the questionnaires in this book, but was willing to spend hours reviewing, revising, and polishing them, no matter how long it took.

The excellent staff members at the American Cancer Society, the American Lung Association, the American Heart Association, the American Diabetes Association, the National Osteoporosis Foundation, and the National Women's Health Network provided background information, resources, and the names of experts to contact.

Jeffrey Stern, M.D., of Waterbury, Connecticut, encouraged me to write this book and acted as my medical consultant. He offered me his wide breadth of medical knowledge as well as his characteristic good humor.

My sincere thanks go to the many women who shared their struggles, and their triumphs, with me. All of the women whose medical cases are described in this book are real, although many names were changed. They were eager to share the most personal details of their lives; their sole concern was that their stories help other women. Without these women this book would not have been written.

FOREWORD

THESE days a woman must act in partnerhip with her physician. But despite all the talk about the partnership between physician and patient, there is often a great gap in communication. This problem may stem from using a different language: medical jargon vs. plain English. It may stem from the lack of time on the part of the physician or from the way the questions are asked by the patient. With the progressive technological advances it is understandable that many physicians concentrate on maintaining and delivering procedures with the goal of improving the patient's health, but too often don't have the time to provide the explanations, counseling, and communication that goes along with it.

Too often the woman may be left consulting the Internet or other sources which she may or may not accept as authoritative or tailored to her needs. This communication gap is especially marked when the questions are related to prevention. Preventative services are not just mammograms, Pap smears, and blood-pressure measurement, but also involve determining a woman's risk factors and building upon them a strategy for avoiding disease.

Risk factors play a key role in numerous critical health care decisions. Whether or not to undergo genetic testing for breast cancer, to use hormone replacement therapy, or when to begin undergoing screening tests for such diseases as colon cancer, diabetes, and osteoporosis are just some examples which underscore the importance of a woman's knowing her risk factors.

This unique book focuses on how to evaluate risk factors and use them in creating a personal health strategy. Charlotte Libov offers the latest information on the prevention of breast, cervical, colon, lung, ovarian, and skin cancer, as well as heart disease, diabetes, osteoporosis, and stroke. In addition, she provides up-to-date advice on quitting smoking, healthful eating, exercise, and hormone replacement therapy. Her guide both explains the importance of risk factors and puts them into perspective, so you can work together with your physician to help beat your risk factors for the common illnesses that threaten the American woman on the brink of the twenty-first century.

I recommend this book highly for every woman who truly wants to become a partner in her health care and improve her personal odds against these common illnesses.

—Lila A. Wallis, M.D., M.A.C.P.

Part One

UNDERSTANDING THE ODDS

CHAPTER 1

YOU CAN CONQUER THE ODDS

IT'S VIRTUALLY IMPOSSIBLE to get through a day without hearing something about our health, whether it's on television, on the radio, in the newspaper, or on the Internet. Often, it seems, it's news of a study which brings information that conflicts with what we just heard about the week before. Instead of helping us to make decisions about our health, this avalanche of often conflicting news is apt to leave us feeling frustrated and confused.

Take Martha, for example. Usually she's bubbly, but the other day she was unusually subdued. "I'm worried I may develop osteoporosis. This morning I saw a television report that it's reaching epidemic proportions," she said.

But Martha has risk factors that should overshadow her concerns about osteoporosis. It's diabetes, not osteoporosis, that runs in her family. She's 40 pounds overweight and doesn't find the time to exercise. Given these risk factors, it's more likely that she'll develop diabetes. But because a new drug for osteoporosis had been approved by the government that week, the disease was in the news. Diabetes, which is deadly and preventable, wasn't in Martha's thoughts. By focusing on osteoporosis, for which she was at low risk, she overlooked steps she could take to prevent diabetes, her more likely threat.

Even though we're swamped with information, there's precious little to help us put it into perspective and extract what we can effectively use. Information is not enough—*you need to know how this information applies to you.*

WHAT THIS BOOK IS

This book is designed to provide you with the information you need to safeguard your health. The focus is on prevention—prevention of the most common and dire diseases that we as women are likely to develop as we grow older.

In keeping with this theme, the ten diseases included here were carefully selected. They share one important thing in common; they are disorders you can *do* something about. These diseases can be prevented or, by being diagnosed earlier, can be better managed or even cured.

To start off, following are some general guidelines to help you understand and assess the information that comes your way, both in this book and from other sources.

RISK FACTORS

To conquer the odds of developing the deadly diseases included in this book, you need to know your risk factors.

A *risk factor* is an independent factor that increases the likelihood of disease. Your family medical history may constitute a risk factor. So may what you eat or how much exercise you get. The environment in which you live or the setting in which you work may also be risk factors. When you know your risk factors, you can create your personal risk profile. This will give you information about the diseases for which you're the most vulnerable, and help you decide what changes, if any, you should make.

In general, risk factors are based on genetics or lifestyle. That is why a sizable portion of this book deals with genetics. However, your heredity is not the only component that determines your well-being.

In fact, when it comes to aging, heredity plays a surprisingly small role—only about 30 percent, according to the MacArthur Foundation Consortium on Successful Aging. Their findings suggest that a whopping 70 percent of the effects of aging are determined by factors in your lifestyle, including what you eat, whether or not you exercise, and your network of social support. This puts most of the control in your hands.

You also need to know about risk factors to help your doctor keep you healthy. Physical examinations used to take over an hour. Nowadays, they may take as little as 15 minutes. The responsibility of knowing more about your health falls upon you. If you know your risk factors, you can ask your doctor for the appropriate referrals, request certain screening tests, and find help to make important lifestyle changes.

As with life, though, this book comes with no guarantee. For example, even though we know that smoking causes an estimated 80 percent of lung cancer cases, it isn't known for certain why some non-smokers get lung cancer and some smokers can puff away with seeming impunity. Or why some people with exemplary lifestyles are felled by a heart attack, while others can snack on fat-laden foods, not budging from the couch, and live into their nineties. What we do have is vast knowledge on which risk factors are most likely to lead to disease, and these offer the best blueprint we have for staying healthy.

WHEN EXPERTS DISAGREE

It would be foolish to pretend there is a consensus about all these subjects. Conflicts between medical experts have been around forever; it's just that, as patients, we were kept in the dark. Now that health news is a hot commodity, reporters go after it. Sometimes they get the medical news even before it appears in medical journals. Thanks to all-news cable television and the Internet, word spreads immediately. So when medical experts disagree, we know all about it.

Sometimes in medicine there is a consensus, and it's easy to make recommendations. But where true controversy reigns, this book includes both sides. This seems frustrating; after all, if the experts can't decide, how can you be expected to? On the other hand, if you know both sides, you know the questions you need to ask in order to make the best decision.

BE A DISCRIMINATING CONSUMER

By its nature, medical news is never-ending. This book contains references to lots and lots of research; yet even as you read it, you'll no doubt be hearing about still more studies. Be discriminating about what news you heed.

For example, here's a sampling of headlines from newspaper articles that appeared within a few weeks:

"Obese People Tend to Lie about Food Intake"
"Study Seeks to Prevent Recurrent Strokes"
"Anti-Estrogens Offer Benefits Without Side Effects"
"Stress Hormone Levels Reduced in Women Who Breast-
    feed"

Since we are constantly assailed by more health information than we can absorb, here are some questions to ask yourself:

- *Is the news useful?* Just because a study has been published doesn't necessarily mean it has useful information for you.
- *What is the relevance of this news report to me?* You can use your risk factors and knowledge of your health and lifestyle to determine this.
- *Have I read the whole article?* Don't just read headlines, or even the first few paragraphs. Important information may be tucked further down.
- *If the medical news is based on study results, what kind of study is it?*

There are basically three different types of studies: experimental, epidemiologic, and clinical.

Experimental studies are usually animal studies, which are preliminary and need to be verified later using human subjects before determining if the findings are relevant at all.

Epidemiologic studies make observations from a given group of participants over time, but do not involve any intervention, or the taking of any action.

Clinical studies are used to back up epidemiologic studies before firm conclusions can be made or an intervention made. In terms of evaluating studies, it is the clinical studies that often contain the "final" word so many of us are seeking.

Other questions to ask about medical studies include:

- *Where is the report published?* A handout in a health food store, for example, may quote a summary of a study done in Europe that may sound good, but there's no way for you to verify it.
- *Was the research done using people like you?* A few years ago, a study done using Finnish men made headlines as to the role of iron in American women. Some important questions were raised, including the differences in genetics, diet, and gender between Finnish men and American women, to name just a few.
- *Is this the first time these results have ever been reported?* If so, it will take awhile for studies to be done to back it up. Also, just because news is billed as a breakthrough doesn't make it so. Many so-called breakthroughs are forgotten about years, or even months, later.
- *Are the statistics meaningful?* Several years ago, a study was done in which patients with pancreatic cancer were asked how much coffee they drank. Although a significant number of coffee drinkers had developed pancreatic cancer, it turned out that coffee had no connection with their disease. Furthermore, bear in mind that statistics refer to groups, not individuals. A study may find that, statistically, reducing cholesterol lowers the risk of a heart attack, but it doesn't guarantee that by reducing your own cholesterol level, you'll avoid a heart attack.
- *Where did the study appear?* Peer-review journals, which are medical journals that don't print studies until they are reviewed

by experts in the same field, are given more credence than other publications. Examples include the *New England Journal of Medicine*, the *British Medical Journal*, the *Journal of the American Medical Association*, and *Lancet*. Other noted journals include those published by the American Heart Association, the American Cancer Society, and the National Cancer Institute.

• *Who sponsored the study?* These days, research that appears in medical journals is sometimes sponsored by private businesses, which can range from drug manufacturers to candy companies. This doesn't necessarily negate the value of the research, but such studies may not tell the whole story. For instance, a study on a drug sponsored by a particular manufacturer may not include alternatives. A study by McDonald's that found that eating an occasional fast-food hamburger wasn't harmful didn't evaluate the impact on people who eat them constantly.

• *Is there a possible conflict of interest?* If the study is of particular interest to you, you can find the original text of it in the journal in which it was published. Many journals are now available in libraries and on the Internet. Look at the author's biographical information to see where the funding for the study came from. Such funding doesn't necessarily indicate bias, but the information does help put the research into perspective. For instance, an analysis published in 1998 in the *Journal of the American Medical Association* found that researchers with funding tied to the tobacco industry more often found secondhand tobacco smoke to be harmless than those who were independently funded.

SCREENING TESTS

Screening tests are one of the most potent tools in diagnosing disease earlier. However, what they do—and don't do—is often misunderstood.

We're very accustomed to getting screening tests, like Pap smears, mammograms, and even community blood-pressure checks. So you may wonder why there aren't screening tests to check for other dangerous diseases.

Developing a useful screening test is complicated. The ideal function of a screening test is not only to diagnose disease early but also to decrease the rate of death from it. Not all screening tests meet this tough standard. For example, chest X rays can detect lung cancer, but they aren't generally considered useful for screening because by the time the tumor is found, it is likely to be incurable. This isn't the case with Pap tests or mammograms, where earlier detection can result in remission or a possible cure.

Throughout this book you will find discussions of various screening tests. Some have proven their worth; others are recommended only for women at higher-than-average risk for a disease; still others remain the subject of debate. Bear in mind that a screening test, like any other medical procedure, can have ramifications, such as possibly leading to unnecessary surgery. So risks and benefits must be weighed.

Advocacy organizations also sometimes disagree over the value of screening tests, such as the clash of opinions over when women should get their first mammograms. To Dr. Barnett Kramer, associate director of the early detection program for the National Institutes of Health (NIH), such disagreements are inevitable. In many countries, he notes, women are given their first mammogram at the age of 50. Here, however, the question of when to have a first mammogram was, up until a few years ago, the topic of vociferous debate. The American Cancer Society recommended that women begin getting regular mammograms at the age of 40. The NIH recommended the age of 50. Ironically, as we learn more about disease such conflicts over screening tests will probably increase.

WARNING SIGNS

This book is designed to be a tool for prevention—to be read before, and hopefully help prevent, the onset of disease. However, information is also included on warning signs. *If you are experiencing such warning signs, don't confuse them with risk factors: take heed and contact your doctor.*

Remember, no book can guarantee that you can conquer the odds of a specific disease. But by paying attention to your risk factors, making changes in your lifestyle, and getting screening tests, you will be doing a vast amount toward conquering the odds.

2

YOUR FAMILY MEDICAL HISTORY: THE GENETIC CONNECTION

LINDSEY'S DOCTOR SCOFFED when the 34-year-old asked him if her chest pain might indicate heart disease. " 'You're too young,' he told me. But my dad had bypass surgery, I'd just lost an uncle to heart disease, and so many people in my family have it that I knew I had to get to the bottom of it," she said.

After she was repeatedly brushed off by her doctor, Lindsey went to see a cardiologist at the Cleveland Clinic Foundation. Tests showed her arteries were becoming narrowed by coronary heart disease. Lindsay followed their recommendations, which include a cholesterol-lowering drug, exercise, and a low-fat diet.

"I go to a step aerobics class three times a week, and I've learned I can't have pizza every night. I know now I have to take this seriously," she says.

If Lindsey hadn't heeded the warnings in her family's medical history, she very well might have suffered a heart attack. But Lindsey is not unusual; everyone's family medical history can yield important clues.

We're all familiar with our family's medical history—or at least we think we are. You go for a checkup, and the doctor asks a few cursory questions about your parents and grandparents. But now that we're learning how much heredity can influence disease, that's not enough anymore. When it comes to genetics, family medical history is being cast in a whole new light.

"In the past," notes Dr. Robert Greenstein, director of the University of Connecticut Health Center's division of human genetics "doctors would take medical histories, but they didn't necessarily take family histories which could recognize patterns suggesting genetic disorders passed down from family member to family member. The doctor wouldn't ask much about your family history unless he said, 'Is there anything in your family history that you think I should know?' " That's not enough, since "your family medical history is the nuts and bolts of your life."

Knowing your family history can:

• Reveal your risk for a particular disease
• Indicate if a genetic birth defect may run in your family
• Provide you with motivation to make needed lifestyle changes to reduce your risk of disease, such as quitting smoking or getting more exercise.

In some cases, learning what happened to your relatives can save your life.

Consider author Carol Krause. Following the death of several of her relatives from cancer, Krause traced her family tree and discovered a deadly inherited cancer syndrome. Because she had this information, she and her sister underwent tests, and their cancers were caught early. "My sisters and cousins know it is our medical family tree that has given us all a chance to live," writes Krause in her book, *How Healthy Is Your Family Tree?* (See Resources section.)

Often, though, potential problems aren't clear-cut. For example, you might assume that a woman whose mother suffered a heart attack at the age of 55 has heart disease in her family. But that isn't necessarily the case if the mother was a heavy smoker. So lifestyle needs to be factored in as well. Still, your family medical history is your best window into your genes.

Here is an example of the family medical history portion of a doctor's exam. You should know the answers to these questions *before* you see your doctor.

The following questions are about your family's medical history (parents, grandparents, and siblings):

Is there a history of heart disease?	Yes____	No____
Is there a history of high blood pressure?	Yes____	No____
Is there a history of diabetes?	Yes____	No____
Is there a history of high cholesterol?	Yes____	No____
Is there a history of gout?	Yes____	No____
Is there a history of kidney disease?	Yes____	No____
Is there a history of kidney stones?	Yes____	No____
Is there a history of stroke?	Yes____	No____
Is there a history of seizures?	Yes____	No____
Is there a history of asthma or hay fever?	Yes____	No____
Is there a history of thyroid diseases?	Yes____	No____
Is there a history of migraine headache?	Yes____	No____
Is there a history of cancer?	Yes____	No____
Is there a history of bowel diseases?	Yes____	No____
Is there a history of ulcer disease?	Yes____	No____
Is there a history of autoimmune diseases such as rheumatoid arthritis or lupus?*	Yes____	No____
Is there a history of depression or other psychiatric disorders?	Yes____	No____
Is there a history of alcohol abuse?	Yes____	No____
Is there a history of neurologic diseases?	Yes____	No____
How many brothers and/or sisters do or did you have?		

*An autoimmune disorder occurs when the body's autoimmune system goes awry, attacking its own cells and tissues.

These questions are designed to facilitate discussion with your doctor about your family medical history and can serve as a starting point to chart your family medical tree (see chapter 3).

IT'S ALL IN YOUR GENES . . . OR IS IT?

Look in the mirror, and you can see how your appearance reflects your heredity. Similarly, your family medical history can be a mirror of the inner workings of your body.

Genetics is the field of biology that has enabled us to make sense of heredity, the transmission of characteristics from parents to offspring. Here's a brief look at how heredity works.

The cells of our body contain an estimated 100,000 genes, which determine such traits as our hair and eye color, how our bodies are built, and possibly even some of our personality characteristics. The genes are wound around lengthy strands of DNA (deoxyribonucleic acid), the molecule that encodes heredity information, and packed into 23 pairs of chromosomes, which are threadlike structures in our cells.

The only cells in the human body that don't have 23 pairs of chromosomes are the sperm and egg cells, which have 23 single chromosomes each. At conception, when the egg and sperm unite, this creates the 23 chromosomal pairs needed for a new human life. Therefore, each of us is conceived with a unique genetic blueprint, half contributed by each of our parents.

The DNA that resides within the genes contains the genetic code that oversees the manner in which our cells function. But occasionally a mistake, or genetic mutation, can occur. This can happen in three ways:

- A mutation can occur when the egg and sperm are forming.
- A mutation can be inherited.
- A gene can be damaged by exposure to an environmental factor.

But even if a gene mutation is inherited, that's no guarantee that a disease or disorder will result. Genes come in two varieties: dominant and recessive. Dominant genetic mutations, such as the one that causes Huntington's chorea, a degenerative nerve disease, only need to be inherited from a single parent to produce the effect. Thus, there's a fifty-fifty chance that a child born of a parent who carries the gene for this disease will inherit it. Recessive genes, such as the mutation that produces cystic fibrosis, an inherited lung disorder, must be inherited from both parents to produce the trait, so the chance that a child will inherit such a gene when both parents carry it is only one in four. A parent can pass on a genetic mutation, but it may not show up, or be expressed, until later generations.

Once genetic mutations were thought responsible only for rare ailments such as Huntington's and cystic fibrosis, which are directly inherited. But scientists have discovered genetic links for common killers as well, including cancer, heart disease, and diabetes. Although these are not inherited diseases in the strict sense of the word, the tendency to develop them may very well be. However, the connection is more complicated to determine because these diseases probably result from complex interactions among several genes.

A particularly important area of genetics focuses on birth defects. If you are pregnant or considering having children, learning about your family's medical history is extremely important. For more information on this, contact your local chapter of the March of Dimes.

Although genetics may set the stage for these common killer diseases, whether or not you develop them may be influenced by a host of lifestyle factors, including smoking, eating a high-fat diet, exposure to cancer-causing chemicals, and other factors yet to be identified. So if you may have inherited a susceptibility gene, you still can change other factors to lower your risk. For example, you may be born with a predisposition to develop diabetes, but by staying lean and physically active, you may be able to avoid developing it.

WHAT GENETICS CAN—AND CANNOT—TELL YOU

Our current knowledge of genetics and disease comes from a $3 billion research program known as the Human Genome Project.

This project's goal is to completely map all the genes in the human body and learn how they interact. This knowledge, it is hoped, will enable doctors to correct genetic mutations, transforming the field of medicine.

For a while it seemed that new genetic discoveries were being made almost daily. Indeed, it's hard not to get carried away with the possibilities and envision a day when we're able to waltz into our doctor's office, relinquish a bit of cellular tissue, and receive a computerized printout of all the diseases to which we are prone. But that day is not yet here.

Indeed, genetic testing is not without its drawbacks.

Although a woman may be able to learn through genetic testing that she has inherited a genetic mutation, it isn't known with certainty whether or not she'll develop the disease. Even if she falls into the very highest risk category for inherited breast cancer, this doesn't mean she has a hundred percent chance of getting the disease. Thus she is faced with a difficult array of choices, ranging from "watchful waiting" to having her breasts removed as a precautionary measure.

Furthermore, as genetic testing becomes more common, there is a concern that not enough emphasis will be placed on providing psychological support for the women who do carry gene mutations, or even for those who learn they don't and feel guilty about it if other family members are afflicted. Another important aspect is the fear that those found to carry a genetic mutation could potentially lose their health insurance or face other forms of discrimination.

With all the attention being focused on genetic testing, the importance of simply knowing your family medical history is easily eclipsed. But this history is important. You may uncover a potentially dangerous genetic disease. Such knowledge could save your life. More likely, what you learn about your family's medical history will not be so dramatic, but it will furnish important clues that can help you conquer the odds.

3

MAPPING YOUR
FAMILY MEDICAL TREE

YOUR FAMILY MEDICAL TREE can be as simple or as elaborate as you like, as long as it contains all the information you need.

This book covers the diseases which afflict most women. However, you can tailor your family medical tree to trace other problems, such as rare genetic diseases, birth defects, or mental illness. (Also, if you decide to get involved more deeply in genealogy, the Resources section lists additional tools.)

As you go about gathering information from your family, be tactful. Often people don't relish talking about death or disease. Guilt can also play a role; no loving parents want to believe they may have, however inadvertently, passed down a harmful trait. Sending your relatives a written questionnaire may be preferable; that way they can fill in exactly the information you need. Don't overlook relatives who died young; such deaths may be a tip-off to an inherited malady.

Get the most specific information possible. Use death certificates and medical records to double-check. A term like *heart trouble* can refer to numerous ailments, only some of which have genetic implications. You may also have to dig deeper when tracking family cases of cancer. Not so long ago, discussing cancer was virtually taboo, says

Dr. Larry Norton, head, division of Solid Tumor Oncology and director of the Evelyn H. Lauder Breast Center at the Memorial Sloan-Kettering Cancer Center.

"If you go back a generation, people didn't talk about breast cancer or ovarian cancer. You would take a history and ask, 'Did you have any breast cancer in your family,' and they'd say no. Then you'd say, 'Well, let's just go through it,' and it would turn out that the mother died of bone cancer and her sister died of liver cancer. But what had really happened was that both had breast cancer; one's had spread to the bone and the other's to the liver. So you need to dig a little bit," says Dr. Norton. As he notes, when it comes to cancer, the important fact to learn is where the cancer originated, not where it spread.

How wide a net should you cast, and how far back should you go? Include as many relatives as you can, so you can uncover trends. "Most people can trace a few dozen people at the most, but families extend into the hundreds. If you go back three or four generations and map out all the connections, you'll find you have a very large family," Dr. Norton says.

Especially in the case of cancer, don't discount the clues that more distant relatives, like cousins, can provide. For instance, Rhonda was concerned that she had inherited a breast cancer gene but was unaware of any other potential problems. She brought her cousin along to the counseling session. Thanks to information the cousin revealed, it turned out both women were at increased risk for ovarian cancer, a fact neither one had realized.

WHAT IF YOU ARE ADOPTED?

Everyone has a family medical history, but if you're adopted, you may have no knowledge of yours. This is a difficult situation.

Ellen, at 51, has been searching for years to locate her biological parents. Recently she learned that her biological mother died of ovarian cancer. Now, to learn more, Ellen is searching for a sister whose existence she just discovered.

"All women who are adopted have no family medical history. We are at risk for everything; you just don't know," says Ellen.

Not knowing what your family medical history is can hold important ramifications for your own health, but whether or not to begin a search for your biological parents is a personal choice. However, you may be able to obtain information on your biological parents' medical history without their identities being revealed. If you know the name of the adoption agency that placed you, write and ask what procedure to follow. If you don't know that information, contact the Adoptees Liberty Movement Association, listed in the Resources section, to learn how to begin a search.

MAPPING YOUR FAMILY'S MEDICAL TREE

1. Make a list of your relatives. Divide your relatives into these categories:

First-degree relatives: Parents, brothers, sisters, and children

Second-degree relatives: Grandparents, aunts, and uncles (we receive one-quarter of our grandparents' genes)

Third-degree relatives: First cousins and great-grandparents

2. Construct Your Family Medical Tree.

Your names, and the names of your brothers and sisters, go on the bottom. On the row above, put your parents' names, as well as their siblings. The names of your four grandparents go on the top line. Such charts usually put male relatives in squares and female relatives in circles, and indicate marriages by connecting relatives with horizontal lines.

3. Record the birth, date of death, and cause of death of each relative who has died.

If your family isn't forthcoming, or your relatives simply don't know, request a death certificate from the health department in the state where the person died. You may also be able to obtain information from relatives' medical records or hospitals where they died. Birth and death certificates are also sometimes tucked into family Bibles.

4. Record all major illnesses and major surgeries.

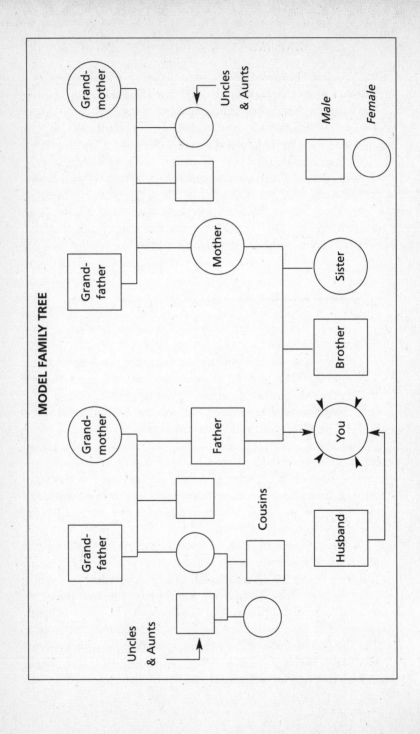

MODEL FAMILY TREE

It isn't only the medical history of relatives who died that you should be concerned about; diseases that affect those who are living can also provide useful information.

5. Be certain to include the ages of your relatives when they died or were diagnosed with their ailments.

Generally, the earlier a disease occurs, the more likely it is that genetics played a role, so knowing the ages involved can help distinguish whether it was heredity or simply aging at work.

6. Record lifestyle factors that may have contributed to illness.

Smoking, obesity, and alcohol and/or drug abuse are some of the factors that can cause diseases that at first may appear to be part of an inherited trend.

7. Record occupations if pertinent.

Exposure to asbestos or other toxic chemicals can cause illness or death.

8. Record unusual physical characteristics.

Check the family photo album; sometimes the way people look can indicate physical problems. Marfan's disease, a rare inherited connective-tissue disorder, causes people to grow tall and thin, with long, spidery fingers and a deformed chest and spine. Overweight people are more likely to have coronary heart disease or diabetes. If your grandmother had a dowager's hump, she probably had osteoporosis.

Now that you've constructed your family medical tree, here's how to "read" it.

• Pay the most attention to your mother's and father's medical histories. They each contributed half of your genetic blueprint. You inherited most of your genes from them, less from your grandparents, aunts and uncles, and less still from your great-grandparents.

• Pay attention to both sides of your family. With "female" diseases, such as breast cancer or ovarian cancer, don't assume that only your mother's side of the family tree is important. While the mother's genetic history is usually the most significant, your father could carry a genetic defect, and the cancer could reveal itself in the medical history of your father's grandmother, mother, sisters, or cousins.

• Look at age. The earlier a disease develops, the more likely it is that heredity was involved. If a family member develops a disease significantly earlier than it affects most people, for example, your mother developed heart disease in her late forties, or your father was diagnosed with it in his late thirties, that may be a tip-off that heredity may be involved.

• Look for clusters. A bunching of cases of the same disease on one side of your family tree is more suggestive that genetics is involved.

• Bear in mind that it's quite likely you won't discover any obvious genetic patterns. But don't overlook sporadic cases of what may be "susceptibility" diseases, those which aren't directly inherited but which you are more likely to develop because of your genetic makeup, such as heart disease and diabetes. This can give you important information about lifestyle factors you must change.

• Consider genetic counseling, if warranted.

This chapter provides information you can use informally to evaluate your risk of the diseases covered in this book. However, if you become aware of a potentially dangerous pattern of an inherited disease, discuss it with your doctor or contact a genetic counselor. Typically, genetic counselors hold a master of science degree in genetics and are certified by the American Board of Genetics. Your doctor can probably refer you to one, or you can contact a major hospital or medical center, or check Resources, page 322.

Either of these two factors may indicate the need for genetic counseling:

1. Two first-degree relatives with the same type of cancer. Breast, uterine, ovarian, and colon cancers should be considered the same because they may stem from a single genetic defect.

2. One first-degree relative under the age of 50 who has an illness usually associated with older people, such as cancer or coronary heart disease.

Remember, genetics is a complex science, and these red flags do not necessarily mean heredity is involved.

Beat Your Risk: If your family medical tree turns up a potentially dangerous trend, don't panic, but do consult a professional genetics counselor. Just on the face of it, such a history can be misleading. You may decide that you want to undergo genetic or diagnostic testing, or you may learn that there is no cause for concern. But at least you'll have the facts.

CANCER RISK SCREENING CLINICS

Throughout this book you'll find mention made of high-risk cancer screening clinics. These programs, established to identify and evaluate those who are at genetically higher-than-average risk of cancer, are springing up all over the country. They are designed to offer several services for people deemed at higher-than-average cancer risk, all under one roof.

These clinics can help clients reasonably evaluate their risk of cancer. Sometimes the risk is lower than you expect it to be, especially if you've had relatives who died from cancer. Dr. Patrick Borgen, who directs the Special Surveillance Breast Project at Memorial Sloan-Kettering, said that when 100 women, each with one family member who had breast cancer, were asked to evaluate their own risk, they pegged it far higher than genetic testing later proved it to be.

It is hoped that the regimen of screening tests offered by these programs results in detecting cancers earlier. According to Dr. Borgen, a study found that 95 percent of the cancers discovered in his program's participants were at a "small and potentially curable" state, while such early cancers were found in only 75 to 78 percent of the women who came to the hospital for other reasons.

Furthermore, such programs can provide enrollees with access to research trials in genetic testing and treatment that may not yet be generally available.

If you are considering such a program, bear in mind that its cost may not be covered by health insurance. Even if it is, you may not want to use it because of the concern that health insurers may use the findings to deny coverage to those found to be at risk.

THE BOTTOM LINE

No matter what your family medical tree turns up, remember that *heredity is not necessarily destiny*. Someone with seemingly little to worry about genetically can undo that fine family medical history by smoking or abusing alcohol. On the other hand, even if your family history seems stacked against you, the choices you make can help you beat your risk factors.

4

CONQUERING CANCER: THE BASICS

MORE THAN 500,000 WOMEN are diagnosed with cancer each year, and more than 250,000 die annually of the disease. Cancer is our country's number two killer and is inching up to number one.

More than a quarter of a century ago, President Richard Nixon signed a bill declaring America "at war" with cancer. Back then it was naively assumed that any country that could put an astronaut on the moon could find a cure for cancer. How wrong we were!

Still, dramatic strides against cancer have been made. Most of this progress has come in the form of knowledge, as we now know more about cancer than ever before. We know it is not a single disease but scores of different types. Some of these remain the biggest killers of women, including lung, breast, and ovarian cancer.

This book covers different types of cancers, all with different characteristics. But they share many similarities. This chapter highlights these similarities and will increase your knowledge of cancer so that you can better use the specific cancer-conquering information contained in the rest of this book.

WHY LEARN ABOUT CANCER?

The subject of cancer used to be shrouded in ignorance. Indeed, the very word cancer was not uttered; the disease was so frightening it was referred to only as the C-word. Cancer is still often equated with a death sentence. It can be, but millions of Americans living today are cancer survivors. It's important to recognize this, because fear of cancer often prevents people from seeking help. If you are paralyzed with fear, you won't practice the steps you need to conquer it. You won't do the self-exams or screening tests, or pay attention to the warning signs—all the actions that result in cancer being detected early and cured.

WHAT IS CANCER?

Although we tend to speak of it as a single disease, cancer is actually an umbrella term encompassing at least a hundred different diseases and maybe more. Here's a simplified explanation of what happens when a cancer occurs.

As you'll recall, almost all of the cells of our body contain genes, composed of DNA, which orchestrate the cells' functioning. Scientists now understand that the changes which cause cancer occur deep within the cellular DNA. The DNA is responsible for programming all the cells in your body to live for a specific period of time. When this occurs normally, the cells multiply, divide, and die in an orderly fashion. But when a normal cell mutates into a cancerous cell, it becomes, in essence, immortal. The cell stops responding to the DNA's growth-inhibiting signals and replicates unceasingly. These cells also gain the ability to "metastasize," or spread, and establish colonies in distant organs, which become tumors. These two cellular characteristics—the ability to grow uncontrollably and to spread—are the hallmarks of a cancer.

Thus, scientists now understand that cancer is a genetic disease. The cancer-causing genetic changes can occur as the result either of a genetic mutation inherited from the parents or of something that occurs during one's lifetime to damage this genetic material, such as exposure to tobacco smoke or other cancer-causing toxins.

Although it is believed that all cancers are linked to genetic defects, the impact varies. Some cancers are thought to be directly inherited—they are linked to a specific gene that may be passed from one generation to another. Five percent of all breast cancer genes are believed to be directly inherited in this way. A larger class of cancers, called *familial* cancers, occur in certain families in higher-than-expected numbers, but they don't follow the normal rules of inheritance. For example, if your mother or brother develops lung cancer, this doesn't mean that you will definitely inherit it. But your risk of developing it is three times that of someone without such a family history.

WHY DO GOOD GENES GO BAD?

The process by which a normal cell undergoes malignant transformation is known as *carcinogenesis*. Sometimes the stage for this process is set before birth; a mutant gene can be inherited from a father or mother, or a defect can occur in a chromosome when the egg and sperm cells unite. But genetic mutations can also occur spontaneously during the process of cell division, or they can be caused by damage from factors in the environment, like cigarette smoke or asbestos, for instance.

In fact, your body has the ability to withstand such damage. The cells of your immune system patrol relentlessly, eliminating potentially cancerous abnormalities. Our biological ability to protect ourselves from cancer varies tremendously from person to person, or even within the same person as we age, and not everyone who inherits a cancer-causing genetic defect develops the disease.

Certain types of genes are linked with carcinogenesis, or the cancer process. These include *oncogenes*, which are genes within the cell that may initiate the cell's transformation from normal to malignant, and *tumor suppressor genes*. Tumor suppressor genes are involved in controlling the cell cycle. We are all born with an important tumor suppressor gene, known as p53, which acts by sensing DNA damage within a cell and preventing the cell from replicating until the damage is repaired. If the damage is repaired, p53 allows the cell to divide. If the DNA damage is too extensive, p53 causes the cell to die. However, if there is a mutation in this important tumor suppressor gene which impairs its function, the genetically damaged cells replicate, and the cancerous process is underway. The p53 gene is believed to be implicated in some 50 different types of cancer, but other such genes are also being discovered.

The "two-hit" or "multiple-hit" theory of cancer holds that, in order for a cancer to begin, a gene must suffer more than two "hits." To envision this, picture a set of chromosomes that suppress breast cancer as similar to the two sets of brakes on your car. If you inherit a genetic mutation for breast cancer, this would knock out one set of brakes, but the other pair would hold the cancer in check, like the second pair of brakes that keeps your car from slipping. But if during your life the other chromosome (or brake) is damaged, there is nothing to halt the cancer from occurring (or the car from slipping downhill).

WHAT CAUSES CANCER?

"I get my clothing dry-cleaned. I use computers. I'm thinking of buying a cellular phone. There's no way I can live my life and, at the same time, worry that everything I do will give me cancer," exclaimed Faith in frustration upon spying yet another article purporting that some feature of our modern life may be giving us cancer. Indeed, it may sometimes seem that we're being told that everything around us causes cancer.

Although some causes of cancer have been discovered, much remains unknown. But medical researchers have uncovered some facts to explain some cancers and some important clues for others.

Growing Older

It's devastating when a young person dies of cancer, but this is more often the exception than the rule. Your risk of developing cancer increases as you age. Nationally, 60 percent of all cancers are diagnosed in people age 65 and older. In this same age group occur 70 percent of all cancer deaths. Indeed, the aging of baby boomers explains some of the increase in many types of cancer. Why is this so? It's not known for certain, but it's believed mutations in certain genes become more common as we grow older. In addition, it is believed that as we age our immune systems become less able to prevent these cancer-causing changes from occurring.

Smoking Cigarettes

An estimated one-third of all cancer deaths can be linked to cigarettes. Smoking is the major cause of cancer of the lungs, mouth, pharynx, larynx, and esophagus, but it also contributes to the development of cancers of the pancreas, cervix, kidney, colon, and bladder.

Smokers who also drink excessive amounts of alcohol have an increased risk of cancers of the mouth, larynx, throat, esophagus and liver as well.

Certain Foods and Cooking Practices

Some forms of cancer may be caused by the foods we eat or the ways in which they are prepared. For example, fatty foods and lack of fiber are believed to increase the risk of colon cancer. Fatty foods may also be implicated in causing breast cancer, although the evidence is conflicting. Salt and pickling are associated with high rates of cancer of the esophagus and stomach.

Environmental Hazards

The overall risk of developing cancer has increased dramatically over the past century. Some of these cases can be attributed to an aging population and better detection. But some contend that these explanations fall short, and they've turned their attention to find out if there are hazards in our surroundings that cause cancer. Some potential sites get great interest, such as Long Island, New York, where there is a higher rate of breast cancer than would normally be expected. But linking such factors to cancer in humans is not that simple a matter. Potentially hazardous substances can vary in the level of danger they pose, according to the concentration of the carcinogen in the environment and the amount of exposure received. So it's easy to see why studies examining these factors often arrive at different conclusions.

Chemicals

There are 23 chemicals known to cause cancer in humans: 4-Aminobiphenyl, arsenic, asbestos, auramine, benzene, benzidine, benzo (a) pyrene, beryllium, bis (chloromethyl) ether, cadmium, chromium and certain chromium compounds, coke-oven emissions, iron oxide, isopropyl oil mustard gas, 2-Naphthylamine, nickel, petroleum, polycyclic aromatic hydrocarbons, radiation, radon, ultraviolet rays, and vinyl chloride.

In addition, there are 150 more chemical substances that are reasonably thought to cause cancer. Here is where some of these known and suspected carcinogens are found:

Pesticides

Over the years pesticides have been more tightly scrutinized because of the concern that some substances used in them may cause cancer.

One type of pesticide, the organochlorides, contain substances that researchers believe can act like a weak form of estrogen, known as a *xenoestrogen*, in the body. These chemicals, which include DDT, PCBs, and dioxin, are found in a vast array of products, including some pesticides and lawn-care products, cosmetics, and plastic bottles.

Normally, during puberty, estrogen encourages breast cells to divide by attaching itself to a molecule called an *estrogen receptor* that is located inside breast cells. But, for unknown reasons, estrogen occasionally triggers cell division after puberty, encouraging tumors to form.

Scientists used to believe that few substances other than estrogen could attach to estrogen receptors. But when researchers combined pollutants and breast cells in the lab, some of the chemicals appeared to attach to the receptor molecules just as estrogen does. Thus, they have become known as *environmental estrogen* for their abilities to act like estrogen.

Although DDT was banned years ago, its residue lingers forever. A study published in 1993 in the *Journal of the National Cancer Institute* compared a group of women with breast cancer to those who were healthy. The study found that participants with breast cancer were more likely to contain higher levels of a breakdown product of DDT called DDE in their breast tissue. After adjusting for other risk factors, the study showed that women with these higher concentrations had a fourfold increased risk of breast cancer. However, subsequent studies have found differing results, including one published in 1997 in the *British Medical Journal,* which found that women with breast cancer had body tissue that contained slightly less DDE than healthy women. Still, interest in the potential DDT connection remains high, and studies are currently under way to learn more about how these xenoestrogens affect the body.

Food Additives and Preservatives

Salt and pickling are associated with high rates of cancer of the esophagus, stomach, and nasopharynx. These cancers are rare in the United States but common in China, where salted fish and pickled vegetables are eaten in much larger quantities. Flavor enhancers and preservatives, though, have also been viewed with suspicion. In 1996, a panel from the prestigious National Academy of Sciences took issue with this view, saying that cancer comes not from food additives but "from diets too rich in calories, fat or alcohol."

"While some chemicals in the diet do have the ability to cause cancer, they appear to be a threat only when they are present in foods that form an unusually large part of the diet," wrote committee chair Ronald Estabrook, who heads the biochemistry department at the University of Texas Southwestern Medical Center at Dallas. "The varied and balanced diet needed for good nutrition—including fruits and vegetables—seems to provide significant protection from the natural toxicants in our foods."

This will probably not be the last word on the debate. It is bound to continue as new chemicals are developed and added to the food supply. One such substance is recombinant bovine growth hormone (rBGH), a hormone fed to cows to increase milk production. Although this substance has not been proven to be harmful, some groups are lobbying for special labeling when it is contained in milk and dairy products so consumers will have the choice of whether to purchase it.

Hair Dye

Over one-third of American women use permanent hair dyes, and in the past some chemicals contained in them have been linked to certain cancers. The American Cancer Society decided to find out if there was anything to be concerned about, so a massive study was embarked upon in which ACS volunteers personally queried over half a million women on their hair-dye habits. The findings, published in February 1994 in the *Journal of the National Cancer Institute*, were that permanent hair dye doesn't increase the risk of cancer—with one exception. The study found that women who used black hair dye for more than twenty years increased their risk of two potentially fatal types of cancer; non-Hodgkin's lymphoma, which occurs in the lymph nodes, and multiple myeloma, which affects the bone marrow. This study confirmed earlier studies that had found higher risk of these cancers among such women. However, the study found that only a tiny fraction of women use this type of hair dye over such a long period of time. Because of the design of the study, the research did not establish a cause and effect between permanent black hair dye and this form of cancer, but it is worth keeping in mind if you color your hair.

Electromagnetic Fields

Can electric blankets, television sets, and computer terminals give us cancer? As a society, we've grown increasingly dependent on these devices, but the worry lingers. It is known that ionizing radiation, that is, X rays, can cause cancer. This debate, though, focuses on the non-ionizing radiation of extremely low-frequency electromagnetic fields (EMFs). These fields are created by all electrical currents, from high-voltage power lines to home appliances.

If exposure to ionizing radiation causes cancer, does exposure to non-ionizing radiation do so as well, particularly in the form of EMFs? Some experts are convinced this is so; others, just as vehemently, disagree.

Those who argue that EMFs cause cancer contend that studies have found that people exposed to high levels of EMFs have increased rates of leukemia, brain cancer, and breast cancer. They also point to tests that have found that exposing cells in test tubes to EMFs affects their genetic makeup. Similar changes have been found in laboratory rats, they contend.

But studies involving humans have been conflicting. For example, a 1994 study published in the *Journal of the National Cancer Institute* compared the risk of breast cancer in women who worked as telephone installers, repairers, and line workers. The study found 38 percent more breast cancer cases than would normally occur. However, no excess breast cancer was found in women who worked in seven occupations, such as telephone operators, data keyers, and computer operators, that also involved elevated EMF exposures. Three earlier studies had also found no increased risk. But the scientists urged that more studies be undertaken.

In 1995, the American Physical Society weighed in on the controversy. The organization, which is the world's largest group of physicists, said that after reviewing a thousand papers, they could find no link between EMFs and cancer. However, a year later, a group of British physicists contended that not only does EMF exposure cause cancer, but they had found out why. They maintain that EMFs attract radioactive products of radon, which is known to cause cancer in humans. In 1997 an article appeared in the *Proceedings of the Institute of Electrical and Electronics Engineers* that compared several case studies. The authors stated: "In all of these cases, the evidence in support of links between the fields and cancer is weak and inconsistent. However, in view of the difficulties that are inherent in cancer risk assessment and in proving the negative in general, it is not possible to prove that no such links exist."

Currently, several studies looking at EMF exposure, in everything from electric blankets to cellular phones, are under way. Stay tuned.

WHAT SHOULD YOU DO?

Faced with such controversy, it's very difficult to know what to do. Certainly, it makes sense to avoid substances that are known, or are highly suspect, to cause cancer. But experts who study risk point out that we tend to become more alarmed when we're faced with the new and exotic than with longtime concerns that have become familiar. For example, stories about a pesticide used on apples, Alar, made headlines a few years ago, but that fear has largely evaporated.

This doesn't surprise Dr. Larry Norton at Memorial Sloan-Kettering. "It's not uncommon for a woman to come to see me who is massively obese, doesn't exercise, doesn't perform breast self-exams, and is reluctant to get mammograms, but what she wants to know is 'Should I move out of my neighborhood because they use pesticides?' Compared to the risk of the kinds of things she's doing, the pesticides are a very tiny piece of her total risk."

GUIDELINES IN PREVENTING CANCER

In much of this book, you'll find many specific things you can do to reduce your risk of specific cancers. However, here are some general guidelines:

1. Don't smoke. Smoking is the main cause of lung cancer and accounts for one-third of all cancers.

2. Watch your weight. Excessive weight is linked to some forms of cancer, including colon and breast cancer.

3. Follow these dietary guidelines:

Eat lots of fruits and vegetables. As you'll see later in this book, fruits and vegetables contain scores of chemicals believed to have cancer-fighting properties.

Eat high fiber foods. Whole-grain cereals, vegetables, and fruits that are high in fiber may help prevent colon cancer.

Eat less cured meat. Foods like ham, bacon, bologna, and hot dogs contain nitrates, which can increase the risk of colon and some types of stomach cancer.

4. Exercise. Being physically active reduces the risk of colon cancer and possibly breast cancer as well.

5. Drink alcohol sparingly. Alcohol has been linked to the risk of breast cancer, as well as cancer of the mouth, throat, and stomach.

6. Avoid overexposure to the sun. Sun exposure is a risk factor for skin cancer. Avoid tanning parlors as well.

7. Handle harmful chemicals safely. Avoid carcinogenic chemicals in the workplace and at home; if you must use them, wear protective clothing.

8. Work cancer screening into your schedule. Screening tests are an important way to detect cancer early enough to cure it. Get in the habit of adding screening tests to your to-do list.

These simple habits can reduce your risk of cancer. More specific guidelines, including information on genetics, screening tests, and other factors, are included in each chapter that follows.

Part Two

CONQUERING THE TEN TOP KILLERS OF WOMEN

5

BREAST CANCER

WHEN SHE WAS 41, Betty went for a routine mammogram, and it showed breast cancer. She was stunned. "I have no family history of breast cancer or any risk factors that I knew of. So this came as a total shock to me," she said.

Donna's breast cancer was not a surprise. "There is a lot of cancer in my family. A *lot*. Ever since my mother was diagnosed three years ago, I have thought of it every day. So when I discovered my lump, I scheduled an immediate mammogram, even though many people told me that, at 29, I was too young to get breast cancer. I looked forward to the test, hoping they were right. But they weren't. I did have breast cancer."

Breast cancer is unpredictable. It strikes women who have risk factors but more often those who don't.

Breast cancer is a common disease. An estimated 207,000 women are diagnosed with breast cancer every year (182,000 with invasive breast cancer, capable of spreading, and 25,000 with the noninvasive type). Every year an estimated 43,500 women die from it.

Until 1995 the death rate from breast cancer remained stable. That year it dropped by 5 percent. Although this is not a whopping decrease, it is a sign of hope.

How probable is it that you'll get breast cancer? Probably not as likely as you think. Publicity surrounding celebrities who have developed breast cancer has raised awareness, but it's also given women an unrealistic picture of their risk. Such attention also gives women the mistaken picture that the incidence of breast cancer is increasing. However, after increasing about 4 percent a year in the 1980s, breast cancer incidence rates have leveled off in recent years to about 110 cases per 100,000 women, according to the American Cancer Society.

The prospect of breast cancer is so scary it can be psychologically paralyzing. A woman told she is at *significantly* increased risk interprets that to mean she's a walking time bomb, even though, in statistical terms, significant connotes only a tiny increase. This is especially true of women with relatives who have been diagnosed with the disease, notes Patrick Borgen at Memorial Sloan-Kettering. In a study 100 women, all with one affected relative, were asked to estimate their breast cancer risk. On average, they thought their risk was 75 percent when, in reality, it was 21 percent, he said.

When considering breast cancer, you must keep your head. Only then can you make the choices that are right for you.

For instance, you probably believe that "one in every nine women will develop breast cancer." The figure is intended to show a woman has a one-in-nine chance of developing breast cancer over an 85-year lifespan, but many women misinterpret it to mean they have a one-in-nine chance of developing breast cancer right this instant. The actual risk during most of your life is far less. For instance, of developing breast cancer by age 50, risk is only 1 in 50. By 60, it doubles, to about 1 in 24.

FACTORS THAT INCREASE YOUR RISK OF BREAST CANCER

Growing Older

No matter how old a woman is when she dies of breast cancer, it is a tragedy. However, when a young woman dies, it is also a human-interest story. So the fact that most breast cancer victims are over 60 when they get this disease is overlooked, because breast cancer victims portrayed in the media tend to be much younger. But these women are exceptions. Although one in nine women will eventually develop breast cancer, this is a cumulative risk estimate over a woman's entire lifespan, with half of that risk occurring after the age of 65. Breast cancer risk is rare in younger women, so if you're under the age of 39, your risk estimate is 1 in 227; it is 1 in 25 between the age of 40 and 59, and 1 in 15 between ages 60 and 79.

Race

Breast cancer is common in every major racial group, but there are some differences. About 16,600 African-American women develop breast cancer every year, and about 5,200 die of the disease annually. African-American women under the age of 50 have a higher risk of developing breast cancer than whites but an overall lower lifetime risk of about 40 percent. However, if they do develop breast cancer, they are twice as likely to die from it. There are conflicting findings on whether this is due to the fact that African-American women are more likely to lack access to preventative health care, such as mammography, or whether there is something about the cancer they get that makes it more deadly.

Latina women have a lower incidence of breast cancer than white or African-American women, but those who develop it are, like African-American women, more likely to die. The rate of breast cancer in Latina women is increasing faster than for other women. The rate of breast cancer in Asian American women varies greatly, depending on the group, but ranges from 55 per 100,000 in Chinese women to a high rate of 106 per 100,000 for Native Hawaiian women, similar to the rate in white women.

Family Medical History of Breast or Ovarian Cancer

About 20 percent of women with newly diagnosed breast cancer have a close relative, such as a mother, sister, grandmother, or aunt, with the disease. There is no other type of cancer that has a genetic link this strong.

Therefore, your family's medical history offers the most important clues to the odds of your developing inherited breast cancer, even though the genetic link accounts for only a small number of breast cancer cases. Knowing this history is also the only way you can decide whether you want to undergo genetic testing to learn if you've inherited a predisposition for the disease. Even if you decide against it, your family medical history can offer you important clues. A history of ovarian cancer can be important, as one type of gene mutation can cause both breast and ovarian cancer.

The topic of inherited breast cancer was transformed in the mid-1990s with the discovery of the so-called breast cancer genes, known as the BRCA genes. The variations of this gene, which are also linked with ovarian cancer, are being named BRCA1, BRCA2, and so on. Eventually, researchers believe such genetic mutations will account for all of the inherited cases of breast cancer in this country. However, that's only an estimated 5 to 10 percent at most. However, it may turn out that these gene mutations influence noninherited breast cancer as well.

The identification of these so-called breast cancer genes also has implications for Jewish women. It's estimated that as many as one percent of American women who are descended from the Ashkenazi Jews of eastern and central Europe (the ancestry of the majority of Jews living in this country) may carry this genetic mutation, which can also cause ovarian cancer, although to a lesser degree.

The original statistics regarding these genetic mutations were published in 1995. Since then, the estimates have been revised downward, which means that women found to be carrying these mutations are still thought to be at increased risk, although not as high as was once thought. Part of the reason for the overestimation is that the women in the study were drawn from population samples with a strong family history of breast cancer. Whether this finding of increased risk will hold up in future studies remains to be seen.

Obviously, more work needs to be done in this area before accurate, firm statistics can be gathered. This isn't thought to be the last word either; more than 200 mutations have been identified on the two BRCA genes, and how they impact on disease is still not known.

The Genetic Clues

Here are some clues that you might have a hereditary predisposition to develop breast cancer:

- You have a first-degree relative, such as a mother or sister, with the disease, or more than one such relative.
- There is a multigenerational history (grandmother and mother).
- You have several second-degree relatives, such as grandmothers (but not mothers), aunts, and cousins, with the disease.
- The cancer in the affected relative occurred in both breasts.
- The cancer occurred in the relative at a relatively young age. Cancer in a younger-than-average patient is generally a hallmark of inheritance. However, with the discovery of the BRCA1 gene, it's also been found that some breast cancers occurred in women who were older than expected, casting doubt on this rule of thumb.

Inherited breast cancer may also be tricky to spot in your family tree. In most cases an increased genetic predisposition to cancer shows up in cancer that affects a single organ of the body. But this is not true in the case of the breast cancer gene. It is believed that inheriting the BRCA1 gene also may raise the risk of ovarian cancer, although this may be due to the manner in which the families in these studies were selected. At present, researchers have found that women who inherit this gene have up to an 85 percent lifetime chance of developing breast cancer and a 60 percent chance of ovarian cancer. However, subsequent studies have found there numbers may be too high, and risk is no longer being viewed in such absolute terms. Another, rare type of inherited breast cancer is linked with uterine, colon, and prostate cancer. An even rarer gene mutation puts families at risk for breast cancer, prostate cancer, brain tumors, leukemia, and sarcoma, which is cancer of the connective tissue (such as cartilage), blood vessels or the fibrous tissue surrounding or supporting organs. So when you are charting your family history, note whether relatives in your family have had not only breast cancer but these other types as well.

Breast cancer in your family history can sometimes be a deeply shrouded secret. Just twenty years ago the topic of breast cancer was hush-hush. For instance, Donna was told her mother was wheelchair-bound due to arthritis, but the real cause was breast cancer.

On the other hand, if you don't have a family history of breast cancer, don't assume you're home free. All women are at risk of breast cancer.

Genetic Testing: Pros and Cons

With the discovery of genes that cause breast cancer, a great deal of attention has been focused on the wisdom of genetic testing. If you suspect you may have a genetic predisposition to breast cancer, you may be very tempted to undergo genetic testing. This subject was discussed earlier on pages 15–16. But there are several additional factors related specifically to genetic breast cancer testing that you should bear in mind.

The breast cancer gene is a large and complex one, and there are many places on it where a mutation can appear. Current genetic testing is able to pinpoint whether a woman has the gene an estimated 20 to 40 percent of the time. So if the mutation is found, the woman will know for sure. But if it isn't, that doesn't necessarily mean the mutation is not present. And even if it is present, that's no certainty that the woman will develop breast cancer.

In addition, it's difficult to know which women should be tested. Dr. Francis Collins, director of the National Center for Human Genome Research, noted at the third annual Congress on Women's Health in 1994 that although studies of women with BRCA1 mutations found that many did have affected family members, relatively few had the kind of dramatic family history considered highly suggestive of a heredity cancer syndrome.

The problems raised by genetic testing for breast cancer are not only technical ones. There are enormous medical and ethical implications, he notes. While it is becoming increasing possible to identify women who inherit these mutations, there is no agreement about what to do about the results. For instance, there is disagreement as to whether regular mammograms under the age of 50, even in concert with breast self-exams and physician's breast exams, can reduce the breast cancer death rate for these women. It's not even known, in drastic cases, if preventative removal of the breast will help. It also is not known whether the cancer that arises from these mutations should be treated differently.

As noted earlier, there are also psychological implications involved in such testing, as well as the threat of economic discrimination. For all of these reasons, a number of organizations, including the American Society of Human Genetics, the National Breast Cancer Coalition, and the Advisory Council of the National Center for Human Genome Research, have urged that genetic testing be used only for research and not for commercial purposes.

Beat Your Risk: *Since breast cancer predominantly strikes women, it's common to think about only your mother's side of the family. But you can inherit the genetic mutation that causes breast cancer from either your mother's or your father's side of the family. So when you are considering your family medical history, don't forget your father's side.*

Certain Types of Breast Disease

If you, like about half of all women, have lumpy breasts, or almost any noncancerous breast problem at all, you may have been told you have *fibrocystic disease,* a frightening term that may lead you to assume you are at increased risk for breast cancer. But having "lumpy" or "cystic" breasts is not a risk factor at all, according to Dr. Susan Love, a breast surgeon and author. She calls fibrocystic disease "a meaningless umbrella term—a wastebasket into which doctors throw every breast problem that isn't cancerous."

That said, here are specific breast problems that do increase your breast cancer risk:

Atypical hyperplasia

Although no one knows why, some women develop a few extra cells in the ducts of their breast. If this growth continues and the cells become oddly shaped, this is termed *hyperplasia with atypia* or *atypical hyperplasia*. It is a rare condition that does increase breast cancer risk in women who have it by about one percent a year.

Atypical hyperplasia doesn't form a lump, and it's not found on mammograms. It is usually discovered when a biopsy is done on nearby tissues, possibly to check on a lump nearby. An estimated 30 percent of women have some atypical hyperplasia; it's found in about 3 percent of breast tissue biopsies.

Lobular Cancer in Situ (LCIS)

An estimated 25,000 women are diagnosed with LCIS each year. This diagnosis often causes great alarm, particularly when such a woman is erroneously told she has a precancerous condition. LCIS does denote abnormal cells within the breast, but it does not progress into cancer itself. Instead, it serves as a marker, because studies have shown that women with this condition are at increased risk, ranging from 16 to 27 percent, of developing breast cancer in the future. Treatment of LCIS ranges from "watchful waiting" to a mastectomy.

Ductal Carcinoma in Situ (DCIS)

Also known as *precancer*, DCIS is more complex than LCIS. Unlike LCIS, it does not serve only as a marker; it is a lesion that sometimes can grow into cancer. It rarely forms a lump, but it may cause a soft thickening because ducts in the breast become filled with cells. Dr. Love estimates that about 30 percent of the women with untreated DCIS will go on to develop invasive breast cancer in the following ten years.

What about Fibroadenomas?

Although breast cancer is rare under the age of 30, it is not unusual for young women to develop *fibroadenomas*, or benign breast tumors. These are simple tumors that feel like marbles beneath the breast. In many cases these tumors do not have to be removed, especially if they occur in teenagers. However, in women who are middle-aged or older, fibroadenomas should be biopsied to make sure they are not breast cancer.

Fibroadenomas do not turn into breast cancer, but certain types are now considered a warning that the woman may be at increased risk. Most fibroadenomas, an estimated two-thirds of all cases, are composed simply of an overgrowth of tissue and do not constitute a cancer risk. However, the remaining one-third are "complex" and contain cysts, calcifications, or other microscopic abnormalities. Women with this form are considered to be at three to four times increased risk for developing breast cancer, particularly if they have a family history of breast cancer or benign proliferative disease, a type of cell overgrowth found in tissue adjacent to the tumor.

Beat Your Risk: *If you've been diagnosed as having a fibroadenoma, get a report on the type that it is. If the tumor is a "complex" one, discuss with your doctor what other steps you should take. If you have a first-degree family history of breast cancer, having the tumor removed may be warranted.*

Certain Hormonal Factors

What do the following have in common?

- Experienced your first menstruation before the age of 12
- Experienced menopause after the age of 55
- Experienced your first pregnancy after the age of 30
- Experienced no pregnancy

All these factors involve the amount of estrogen manufactured by your body. When it comes to developing breast cancer, the estrogen your body is naturally exposed to plays a role.

If you experienced your first period before the age of 12 and/or you experienced menopause after the age of 55, both of these factors mean that you've had the hormone estrogen circulating in your body longer than most women. This prolonged exposure to estrogen is believed to increase the risk of breast cancer.

Hormones also play a role in pregnancy and breast cancer risk. According to a 1994 paper published in the *New England Journal of Medicine*, it's suggested that the more full-term pregnancies a woman has had, the lower her risk of developing breast cancer after she turns 45. However, there is also evidence which suggests that the more pregnancies a woman undergoes, the higher risk she has of developing breast cancer under that age. Studies also find that the risk of breast cancer is slightly higher for women who give birth to their first child after the age of 30, or bear no children at all. This may account for the slightly higher rates of breast cancer among nuns and childless lesbians.

Breast-feeding has been thought to protect against breast cancer, but the evidence appears dubious. There had been studies, particularly in other countries, including Mexico, Japan, and China, which found an effect. Also, a 1994 study published in the *New England Journal of Medicine* found that teenage mothers who breast-fed had a slightly reduced breast cancer risk, but for older women there was no difference. However, some major studies have found no protective effect at all. A study published in 1996 in the journal *Lancet* found no relationship between breast-feeding and the risk of cancer. In 1997, researchers at the Harvard School of Public Health also examined data from U.S. women as well as those in several other countries, including Wales, Greece, Slovenia, Brazil, Japan, and Taiwan, and found that breast-feeding had no such effect.

Prolonged Use of Oral Contraceptives

Since hormones play a role in breast cancer risk, researchers have long tried to determine if taking birth control pills, which contain estrogen, raises the risk of breast cancer. Generally, the studies done on oral contraceptives and breast cancer risk have found increased risk for some groups of women but not others. The increases in risk involved younger women or those who took the pills for a long time.

In 1994, the journal *Lancet* reported on a Dutch study that evaluated birth control pill use in 918 breast cancer patients compared to a group of healthy women. They found that beginning oral contraceptives at a young age (before 20) and using them for four or more years increased breast cancer risk. However, women who took them between the ages of 25 and 39 showed no adverse effect. There was, however, an increased risk of women who took them after the age of 39. Since older women are at increased risk of breast cancer, any increase, even if slight, should be taken into consideration, they noted.

A study published a few months earlier in the *Journal of the National Cancer Institute* found similar results. This study found that women under the age of 35 who took oral contraceptives for at least 10 years slightly increased their risk of breast cancer when compared to women who had never used them or used them for only a brief period. The study also found a small increase in breast cancer risk for young women who went on oral contraceptives within five years of experiencing their first period. The researchers speculated that this may be because the young women were taking them at a time when their breast cells were still undergoing changes, magnifying the potential for genetic damage.

But gauging the effect of oral contraceptives on breast cancer risk is not easy. For one thing, oral contraceptives went on the market only 25 years ago, so only now are the women who were among the first users entering the age group in which they become more vulnerable to breast cancer. Also, the amount of estrogen that the pills contain has changed over the years, making comparisons difficult. Furthermore, oral contraceptives are sometimes prescribed for young women experiencing menstrual difficulties, and it's possible that these women may run a slightly increased risk of breast cancer for reasons unrelated to the Pill.

Beat Your Risk: *If you are a young woman contemplating using oral contraceptives, you may want to consider another form of contraception for a few years. If you're older and you've been taking oral contraceptives for many years, you might want to consider going off the Pill. Bear in mind, though, that birth control pills may have some positive effects, such as reducing the risk of ovarian cancer.*

Prolonged Use of Hormone Replacement Therapy

Hormone replacement therapy (HRT) prevents osteoporosis and may sharply reduce the risk of heart disease and potentially other diseases. But prolonged use—five years or more—increases breast cancer risk, a fact that must be taken into account. For more information, see chapter 18.

Smoking

There is evidence that indicates smoking cigarettes may turn out to be a risk factor for breast cancer. Although findings have been contradictory in the past, and there was even some thought that smoking might be protective because of its anti-estrogen effects (in some cases estrogen can promote tumor growth), this has not been proven and, indeed, the opposite may be true.

First, as knowledge of genetics increases, some studies are finding that smoking may pose a breast cancer risk factor for women whose genetic makeup makes it more difficult for their body's cells to become rid of toxins. Additionally, there is evidence that, as the population of women smokers age, a link between breast cancer and smoking may become more evident. Some studies also indicate that the risk posed by cigarette smoke may not be limited only to the smokers themselves; there may be an increased threat due to inhaling the smoke indirectly, through secondhand smoke.

Whether smoking turns out to be a major risk factor or not, it's been established that female smokers who develop breast cancer are less likely to survive. A study done at the Roswell Park Cancer Institute in Buffalo, New York, found that female breast cancer patients who had smoked were more likely to have tumors spread to their lungs. Furthermore, a review of patients at Memorial Sloan-Kettering Cancer Center in New York City found that a woman's chances of surviving advanced breast cancer was most affected by whether or not she had smoked. This was also true of African-American women, regardless of their breast cancer stage.

Possible Additional Risk Factors

Because so little is known about what causes breast cancer, researchers are trying to learn what other factors may be involved. What follows is information on factors that may turn out to contribute to breast cancer risk, although thus far not enough evidence exists to consider them major risk factors.

Environmental Risk Factors

Over the past several years researchers have looked into our environment, such as the air we breathe, the water we drink, and the chemicals to which we are exposed, to determine if any of these factors contribute to breast cancer.

Lending credence to such theories is a study published in 1995 in the *Journal of the National Cancer Institute* that looked at 60 groups of immigrants who moved from Australia to Canada or vice versa. Researchers found that with their migration their risk of dying from breast cancer varied to match their adopted country. Indeed, the study found that most of these women had, within 30 years or less, breast cancer death rates indistinguishable from that of local residents. The risk rose for women who left countries with lower breast cancer rates, but for those coming from countries with higher breast cancer rates, the risk dropped.

Such findings indicate that something associated with the immigrants' new homes influences breast cancer risk. But although the studies are intriguing, the authors cautioned that their research looked only at breast cancer death rates, not the development of the disease itself. They also acknowledged that they don't know why the risk changed from one place to the other.

This study may be an important first step in unraveling environmental factors from that of underlying genetic predisposition. Even if a woman is born with a genetic predisposition to breast cancer, these other factors may determine whether or not she develops it, and understanding them may pave the way for new strategies to prevent breast cancer.

Weight Gain after Menopause

Because obesity is associated with so many other risk factors, it seems logical to assume that being overweight increases the risk of breast cancer. But the influence of excess weight on breast cancer risk is a complex issue, one concerning not only the weight itself but when it is gained and where.

Studies have generally found an increased risk of breast cancer for women who become overweight following menopause. Most studies show the women with the greatest risk are those who pile on the excess pounds around their middle. Such a weight distribution is linked to diabetes and heart disease as well. But what puzzles experts is that overweight young women have less risk of breast cancer. Most studies, though, concur that if a woman can manage to stay thin past menopause, her risk of breast cancer is decreased.

A High-Fat Diet

Women who live in Japan eat a diet much lower in fat than that of American women, and they have a much lower breast cancer rate—but is there a connection? Some experts think so, but research thus far fails to prove it. In 1992 a study published in the *Journal of the American Medical Association* found no link between the amount of fat eaten by the women enrolled in the Nurses' Health Study and their rate of breast cancer. Other studies, including one published four years later in the *New England Journal of Medicine* that examined data drawn from 300,000 women, found similar results.

Many still believe in this theory. They point out that memory can be faulty in studies in which participants are asked to recall what they ate. Also, the supposed "low-fat" diet in these studies contained considerable fat, so that may be the reason for the lack of proof. The Women's Health Initiative, a large-scale study, will attempt to sort this out; however, the findings aren't expected for a few more years.

Other factors might also account for the difference between breast cancer rates in American and Japanese women. Genetic factors may be at work. Also, Japanese women eat a diet rich in soy, which some believe may protect against breast cancer. (See chapter 16 for more information.)

Alcohol Use

There is evidence that drinking alcohol may increase breast cancer risk, although the amount it takes is open to question. For more information, see chapter 16.

Being a DES Mother

Diethylstilbestrol (DES) was a synthetic estrogen that was prescribed mostly for pregnant women in the 1940s and 1950s; it continued to be given until the late 1970s. This practice stopped after it was found to be harmful, but its long-range effects on both mothers who took DES and their daughters have been far-reaching. In terms of breast cancer, mothers who took DES are at increased risk, so if you took this drug, you should discuss this with your doctor. For more information on DES, see chapter 6.

Radiation to the Chest (in Moderate to High Doses)

For the vast majority of women, radiation does not constitute a risk factor. But if you are exposed to a large number of chest X rays as a treatment for scoliosis, an abnormal curvature of the spine, or acne, you may be at increased risk. This is also true if, in your twenties, you underwent radiation for the treatment of Hodgkin's disease, a rare type of cancer.

HOW TO REDUCE THE RISK OF
BREAST CANCER

Don't Smoke

As noted, the evidence on whether smoking cigarettes contributes to breast cancer isn't conclusive but may turn out to be the case. So not smoking is a wise choice.

Cut Your Fat Intake

The evidence linking breast cancer to diet is not as strong as that connecting diet and such diseases as heart disease or diabetes. However, research suggests that what you eat may influence your risk, although by how much is not known.

The evidence of a dietary connection stems from the epidemiological studies, mentioned earlier, that show that in Japan, where women eat a diet very low in fat, the rate of breast cancer is rare.

"There is no question that societies that eat less calories and less fat have lower incidence of breast cancer. There is no question that when they increase their fat and calories they have an increase in breast cancer," notes Dr. Norton at Memorial Sloan-Kettering.

However, since not all studies confirm that a low-fat diet decreases breast cancer risk, perhaps the culprit isn't the overall amount of dietary fat that is bad but the particular type of fat. Bolstering this theory are studies that show that, despite their high-fat diet, women living in the Arctic north and the Mediterranean have a lower rate of breast cancer. People in these cultures get their fats primarily from fish oils or olive oil, which are both unsaturated. A study of Greek and American researchers, reported in 1995 in the *Journal of the National Cancer Institute*, found that women who consumed olive oil at more than one meal a day had a 25 percent lower risk of breast cancer. Among the things the study could not determine, though, was whether the olive oil itself was beneficial or because the oil replaced other types of fat. But such findings have led to the support of a "Mediterranean diet" rich in olive oil.

Eat Lots of Fruits and Vegetables

A potent breast cancer preventative may be no further away than your refrigerator. Eating lots of fruits and vegetables is believed to reduce cancer risk because of the *phytochemicals* they contain. Within this type of chemicals is a class called *indoles*, which may specifically lower breast cancer risk; they are found in cruciferous vegetables, such as broccoli, cauliflower, and brussels sprouts. Preliminary studies with mice indicate that one form of this compound helps prevent abnormal stimulation of the female hormone estrogen, therefore, it's theorized, reducing breast cancer risk. More research needs to be done to learn if this is so in humans as well.

Exercise Regularly

Over the years there's been little encouraging news about how to prevent breast cancer, so it made headlines when a study in the *Journal of the National Cancer Institute*, published in 1994, reported that women who exercised an average of four hours a week during the course of their childbearing years cut their breast cancer rate nearly 60 percent! The study also found that women who exercised just one to three hours a week racked up a reduction of 30 percent.

This was not the first time there was good news about exercise. In the 1980s, Rose Frisch, a geneticist at the Harvard School of Public Health, surveyed 5,398 female college graduates to learn which characteristics corresponded with good health. They discovered that the women who had played team sports had not only a 35 percent lower lifetime risk of breast cancer but a 61 percent lower lifetime risk of cervical, uterine, and other reproductive cancers as well. Researchers speculate that exercise alters the production of the ovarian hormones estrogen and progesterone, which accounts for this beneficial effect.

So there's evidence that exercising when you're young may afford you a lifetime of reduced risk from these types of cancer. But will exercise help if you begin when you're older? Some experts believe so. They note that exercise helps women stay lean, and lean women manufacture a less potent type of estrogen, which also may reduce their risk of cancers, including colon cancer.

Not all the studies point to the benefit of exercise; a study published in 1998 in the *Journal of the National Cancer Institute*, which examined information from the Nurses' Health Study, found that exercise during young adulthood does not decrease breast cancer risk later on. But this study acknowledged that the weight of previous studies does point to a benefit.

Practice Early Detection Procedures

Because of the lack of information on what causes breast cancer, much of the emphasis has been on getting screened for this disease in hopes of detecting it early. The problem is that by the time most breast cancers become detectable, they no longer are truly early stage cancers. Before you can feel a lump or see it on a mammogram, most cancers have been there an estimated eight to ten years. By that time the cancer may already have spread. But that doesn't mean that the cancer isn't curable; a lot depends on how aggressive the tumor is, the strength of the woman's immune system, and the sensitivity of the cancer cells to treatment.

With so much emphasis placed on early detection, a woman may be made to feel guilty if she doesn't find her cancer in the earliest possible stage. This isn't necessarily fair. "If the cancer isn't found at stage one, the patient feels guilty or feels it has to be someone's fault. That isn't necessarily true. There has to be room for bad luck and fate," says Dr. Love.

That said, though, early detection is an important way to help reduce your risk.

BREAST CANCER DETECTION

There are three basic methods of breast cancer screening, and they complement each other. They include checking your breasts ("breast self-exam"); having a doctor check your breasts ("a professional, or clinical, breast exam"); and mammography.

Breast Self-Exams

The American Cancer Society recommends that women examine their breasts every month. Those women who practice self-exams even occasionally are more likely to discover their breast cancers earlier than women who find them by chance. But do you need to go to the extent of a formal breast self-exam, following a particular procedure? Some women prefer a formal procedure, but others may not. Which is right? The American Cancer Society endorses a formal procedure, but Dr. Love contends that what's important is that a woman become familiar with how her breasts feels and not be inhibited from touching them. In that way she can discover a lump or other abnormality, without going through a formal regimen.

"Generally speaking, most women do find their own lumps, whether or not they do breast self-exams. Women tell me they had a feeling something was wrong, so they checked their breast. It's just something that tips them off; not a pain, really, but a sense that something is wrong," she noted.

Although what most women look for is a lump, pay attention to any kind of breast changes in general. Anna, 75, and her friend Rita, 68, can attest to the fact that cancer sometimes manifests itself in a form that is not a lump. Longtime friends, they were diagnosed with different types of breast cancer within a year of each other.

Anna's breast became enlarged and reddened. "I love to eat, so I thought maybe I was just gaining weight," she said. Her daughter insisted she go to the doctor. The diagnosis was inflammatory breast cancer.

Rita's breast cancer was a more common type. "I've always had lumpy breasts, and it's very difficult for me to determine what's what," she said. She had a mammogram in April and got a clean bill of health, but in October she noticed a dimpling in her left breast. "Not a lump; just a dimpling," she said. The diagnosis was breast cancer.

When checking your breasts, here are some tips:

1. Become familiar with what your breasts normally feel like. "What women tell me the most is, 'I have so many lumps I don't know what to feel for,' but if you become familiar with your breasts, that's helpful in sorting out what might connote a problem," says Janet Rose Osuch, M.D., former medical director of the Comprehensive Breast Health Clinic at Michigan State University.

2. Check your breasts monthly, around the same time each month. A few days after your menstrual period is a good time because changes caused by the normal effects of varying hormone levels are less likely. As time goes on, you'll be better able to recognize any changes from previous months.

3. Obviously, when you're examining your breasts, what is usually uppermost in your mind is that you are searching for a lump, either in your breasts or near your underarm. But look also for other possible warning signs, including:

- Thickening that does not match with findings in the opposite breast.
- Breast dimpling (similar to the same sort of indentation you find on your cheek).
- Nipple scaliness.
- Breast discharge. This is often cited as a warning sign, but this can be unnecessarily alarming. If you experience discharge when your breasts are squeezed, that's normal. However, spontaneous discharge, the kind that stains your underclothing, can signal a problem.
- Changes in the nipple. Having an inverted nipple is not unusual. But if a formerly outward nipple changes to point inward, or vice versa, that's a change your doctor should check.
- Any redness of the breast, even if it appears to be an infection. Often that is what it is. But redness can also be a warning sign of a serious type of breast cancer known as inflammatory breast cancer. It's most likely that you have an infection and your doctor will give you antibiotics to clear it up. But this isn't a chance you want to take.
- Any breast pain, particularly in connection with a lump. Breast pain is a common problem and usually does not indicate cancer. However, this general guideline has been misinterpreted, leaving the impression that breast pain is always harmless. Occasionally such pain can indicate a lump beneath the area. All

newly discovered breast lumps—whether painful or not—should be brought to a doctor's attention.

Beat Your Risk: *The vast majority of lumps and breast changes are found to be harmless. But this is not your decision to make. If you notice any of these potential warning signs, contact your doctor immediately.*

How to Do a Breast Self-Exam

1. Stand or sit in front of a mirror with your arms at your sides. Look for any changes in the breast, such as dimpling, redness, or different breast size or shape. Bear in mind that many women do have breasts that are different in size; the tip-off here would be a change in the size that has occurred from one month to the next. Stay in the same position, but look for any change using the mirror. Now put your arms up in the air and do the same thing.

2. Lie on your back, put your right arm over your head, and use your left hand to examine your right breast. Palpate (press with your fingers), using dime-sized circles, moving in ever smaller circles from the outside of the breast toward the nipple. Cover the entire breast.

3. Feel the underarm area.

4. Switch to the other side and do steps 2-3 on that side.

Beat Your Risk: *If you think you've found a lump or another type of abnormality, check your other breast. If you find the irregularity in the same place on the other side, it may be nothing to worry about. But if you don't find such an irregularity on the other side, call your doctor.*

Professional Breast Examination

If you are between the ages of 20 and 40, you should have a breast exam done by a doctor or other health professional every three years. If you are past 40, you should have one done annually.

These exams are commonly done as part of a woman's gynecological checkup. In her book, *Modern Breast and Pelvic Examinations,*

Dr. Lila A. Wallis, clinical professor of medicine at Cornell University Medical College, outlines the type of examination you should expect.

She recommends that it start with the doctor looking at your breasts, checking for skin changes, asymmetry, irregularity, and dimpling. The first part of the exam should be done while you are sitting up, and your arms should be placed in a variety of positions, including above and behind your head. Your breasts should be examined while you are lying down as well. Individual doctors vary in their techniques, but the exam should be thorough.

Professional breast examinations can make a difference, especially in finding lumps in the denser breasts of younger women, which mammography may miss. On the other hand, since mammography can find the smaller lumps that cannot yet be felt, the two methods complement each other.

Beat Your Risk: If you notice anything suspicious about your breast, don't be silent and wait to see if the doctor detects it or if it shows up on a mammogram. Bring it to your doctor's attention.

Mammography

There are a lot of misconceptions about what mammography can and cannot do. Once a breast cancer grows large enough to be felt through the skin, it probably has been growing for several years. A mammogram should pick up a cancer when such a mass is still too small to be felt.

Mammograms are not perfect; they miss an estimated 10 to 30 percent of breast cancers. But in the detection of this too often deadly disease, this is the best weapon we have.

How Does It Feel to Have a Mammogram?

A mammography examination is quite straightforward. Your breasts are positioned and compressed between two plastic plates.

Two X rays are taken of each breast, one from above and one from the side. A physician trained in radiology reads the mammogram to see if there are any suspicious areas.

Remember that mammography is not foolproof. A woman may be falsely reassured by a negative mammogram yet turn out to have breast cancer.

Why do mammograms sometimes fail to detect breast cancer? There are several reasons:

- The mass may be obscured by the overlying dense tissue.
- The picture may not have included the part of the breast where the cancer is.
- The picture may be of poor quality.
- Human error—the person reading the film may make a mistake.

So if you have a lump or other suspicious sign, and your mammogram is negative, it still needs to be checked further. Insist on a biopsy, in which a needle is used to remove a small core of tissue, to make sure that there really is nothing to worry about.

Above all, if you believe something is amiss and your doctor doesn't appear concerned, get a second opinion immediately. It's human nature to want to be reassured, but when it comes to breast cancer, this may not be wise. Even if your doctor counsels waiting, and the problem persists, get a second opinion.

Beat Your Risk: *Whenever you seek a second opinion, find a doctor with no ties to the first. See a doctor who is in a different practice or medical group, and/or affiliated with a different hospital. Doctors who practice together may hesitate to disagree with each other.*

Making Sure Your Mammogram Is Accurate

If you're getting a mammogram, you certainly want to make sure it's done properly and interpreted correctly.

First, as with a breast self-exam, you should have your mammogram done right after your menstrual period. As a 1997 study in the journal *Cancer* showed, mammograms done during the first two weeks of a woman's menstrual cycle are less likely to miss breast cancer than those done during the last two weeks. This is probably due to hormonal changes, which tend to make breast tissue denser during the second half of the menstrual cycle. The study's findings held particularly true for women who were currently on, or had previously taken, oral contraceptives and for women on HRT.

When having your mammogram done, it's important that the test be as accurate as possible. Consider having your mammogram done at a major medical center, or even a cancer center, if possible. These mammograms tend to be consistent in quality, while the mammograms done at smaller facilities tend to vary widely.

The federal Food and Drug Administration requires certification of all mammography machines to insure that they meet national safety and accuracy standards. Does this completely solve the problem of inaccurate mammograms? Not necessarily, since staff expertise can vary widely. But it helps a great deal.

Mammograms are not inexpensive, but they are cheap when you consider that they can save your life. The cost varies from $110 to $225. Some states require private insurers to cover part of the cost. Some hospitals sponsor mobile mammography vans, which often cost less.

For a list of mammography facilities in your area that are accredited, call the American Cancer Society at 1-800-ACS-2345. They can also tell you where you can get free or discounted mammograms.

Beat Your Risk: *After you've had your mammogram, do not assume that everything is fine if you do not receive the results. Call and follow up. Ask for a written report and follow up with your doctor if there is anything you don't understand.*

When Should You Begin Getting Mammograms?

For many years, it's been agreed that women should begin getting regular mammograms in their fifties. Up until a few years ago, there was disagreement on whether screening mammography benefited women in their forties. Since then, though, the agencies involved have revised their thinking, and the general recommendation now is that women should begin having screening mammograms in their forties.

It's worthwhile to look at the arguments behind this issue, because they provide an understanding of the limits of mammography.

Although "fifty" is not necessarily a magic number, there are specific reasons why mammography is less effective when used on younger women.

Screening tests are most useful when they are used on those the most likely to have the disease. If you're under forty, you are more likely to receive an abnormal mammogram that is not cancer but requires further testing, resulting in needless worry and biopsies. The National Cancer Institute estimates that a woman who has a yearly mammogram in her forties has about a 30 percent chance of having one of these false-positive mammograms.

Also, before menopause women have dense breast tissue, making cancer more difficult to detect. About 25 percent of breast tumors are missed in women in their forties, compared with 10 percent of tumors of women who are older.

No matter when you begin having regular mammograms, you should have them done annually, so later readings can be compared to earlier ones. This is how cancer is most often detected. Also, if you're in your forties, having annual mammograms is worthwhile because the tumors appearing in younger women are apt to grow more quickly.

Beat Your Risk: *Remember, mammography is a screening tool for women without a family history of breast cancer or any symptoms. If you find a lump, you should have a mammogram, whatever your age. And you should have the mammogram immediately, not wait until your annual one is due.*

Do You Ever Outgrow the Need for Mammograms?

Generally, no. Since the incidence of breast cancer increases as women age, an annual mammogram should always be part of your health care regimen. Unfortunately, though, studies show that women over the age of 65 are not getting the mammograms they need, and the numbers are even worse for African-American women. Studies also indicate that women in this older age range may not be getting professional breast exams either. So if you fall in this age group (or you have loved ones who do), you should make sure you're getting both a mammogram and a professional breast exam each year.

Mammography and Breast Implants

Over two million American women have received breast implants since the practice began. What is the potential of these implants to cause cancer?

In the 1980s, experiments found that some of the substances used in the covering of these implants may cause tumors in rats. But what about women? Not many studies have been done, and no such link has thus far been found. However, implants make it more difficult to detect early breast cancer on mammograms. Since the purpose of mammography is to pick up early breast cancer tumors before they grow large enough to be felt, it is precisely these tumors that may be missed on women with implants. So if you have breast implants, ask your doctor if you can undergo another type of breast cancer detection test instead, such as magnetic resonance imagery (MRI).

By the way, hormone replacement therapy can also make your breasts denser. This is a cause for concern, since HRT also increases the risk of breast cancer. If you are taking HRT, your doctor may want to use another type of test or make sure the person reading the test is aware of this.

Alternatives to Mammography

Because of the limitations of mammography, there is increasing emphasis on using other, or additional, techniques to improve the rate of detection of breast cancer. Ultrasound, MRI, and positron emission tomography (PET) can all be used instead. They are not used for screening, but they may be preferable to mammography if you have unusually dense breasts, scar tissue, or breast implants.

A technique that uses sound waves, ultrasound is used in women who have dense breast tissue. It is also used as a diagnostic device, to distinguish benign abnormalities, such as fluid-filled cysts, from solid ones. In MRI, high radio frequencies in a magnetic field are used to produce images of the breast; it is currently used more as a diagnostic than a screening device. The PET scan, which relies on the use of a radioactive sugar absorbed by the cells, is also more of a follow-up test of a suspicious mammogram rather than a screening test, because currently this device does not have the power to detect small tumors.

Because breast cancer is so frightening, most women believe they are at higher risk than they actually are. Some women, though, truly are at heightened risk. If you fall into this group, here are three options to consider:

Close Surveillance

Close surveillance is the name given to a regimen of increased screening that, hopefully, will result in early detection if cancer does develop. Usually this regimen entails monthly breast self-exams, an annual diagnostic mammogram, and a professional breast examination at four- to six-month intervals.

An evaluation at a high-risk cancer clinic (see chapter 2), with or without genetic testing, can provide a realistic risk assessment and develop a regimen of close surveillance.

Preventative Mastectomy

Prophylactic mastectomy, the removal of the breasts as a preventive measure, is a controversial topic. Although such a step drastically reduces the possibility of breast cancer, it does not completely eliminate it, because the disease can develop in the remaining tissue and even prove fatal, especially if the surgery has given the woman such a false sense of security that she ignores warning signs.

Obviously, preventative mastectomy should involve great thought, say Malcolm M. Bilimoria, M.D., and Monica Morrow, M.D., whose article on the topic appeared in 1995 in CA—A Cancer Journal for Clinicians. "Prophylactic surgery is never an emergency. It should not be undertaken due to misinformation about risk status or anxiety over the death of a relative or friend," they note.

The Society of Surgical Oncology developed a position paper outlining which individuals for whom preventative mastectomy might be considered, Bilimoria and Morrow also note. These include women whose family history includes not simply relatives who developed breast cancer but also one or more relatives who developed a type suggestive of genetic transmission—that is, they developed cancer in both breasts prior to menopause. Other factors include having breasts with atypical hyperplasia and breasts that are dense, lumpy, and difficult to evaluate with screening tests such as mammography. Until recently, close surveillance and preventive removal of the breasts were the only options offered to these high-risk women. However, with the addition now of tamoxifen, this picture is changing, though more research needs to be done.

Tamoxifen

Until 1998 it was thought that not much could be done to prevent breast cancer. This changed after the results of a government-funded study evaluating the effects of tamoxifen came in. In fact, the study was halted 14 months early because the effects were so dramatic.

Essentially, the study, conducted by the National Cancer Institute, examined 13,388 women who were at high risk for breast cancer and found that the drug cut the risk by 46 percent. This was good news because previously tamoxifen had been used in breast cancer patients only to reduce the risk of reoccurrence. The jubilation was tempered, though, by two factors. First, tamoxifen carries with it an increased risk of uterine cancer. And second, two subsequent studies failed to confirm this major reduction in breast cancer risk.

Tamoxifen, the most widely prescribed anticancer drug in the world, belongs to a class of drugs known as *selective estrogen receptor modulators* (SERMs). This means it is an *anti-estrogen*, that is, it blocks the binding of the hormone estrogen to receptors in the breast.

The study found that the drug's effects differed according to age. Basically, women over the age of 50 (who were most likely to be postmenopausal) derived a greater benefit from the drug, but they were also more prone to potentially fatal side effects, including endometrial cancer and blood clots.

In its description of women at high risk of breast cancer, the National Cancer Institute includes those over the age of 60, on the basis of their age alone. However, such women, if they don't have other risk factors, may want to weigh the issue carefully, as they could be exchanging the risk of breast cancer for endometrial cancer. Tamoxifen also should not be taken by a woman over 50 who has a history of blood clots or who still has her uterus, putting her at risk for endometrial cancer. Younger women who haven't reached menopause shouldn't use tamoxifen if they wish to become pregnant. However, women with a strong family history of breast cancer, who have one of the breast cancer genes, or who have LCIS may benefit from the drug.

Tamoxifen is not the only SERM that blocks estrogen receptors in the breast. It is hoped that other drugs in this class, such as Evista (raloxifen), an FDA-approved treatment for halting bone loss, will provide safer alternatives. This is an area that bears watching in the future.

Beat Your Risk *If you are honestly at very high risk for breast cancer, be aware of who the experts are in the field and where they practice. Have a game plan in the event you develop cancer. This is true not only for breast cancer, but other types of cancer as well.*

THE BOTTOM LINE

Dealing with breast cancer is a very difficult subject, in part because so little is known about what causes this deadly disease. Only a small percentage of breast cancer cases are linked to risk factors; the vast majority occur for no identifiable reasons. Here's a summary of the steps you can take:

- Examine your breasts monthly. Bring any changes you find to your health provider's attention.
- Get an annual breast exam by a health care provider.
- Begin annual mammograms at the age of 40, keeping in mind the limitations of mammography in younger women.
- If you are at high risk for breast cancer, seek expert medical advice to learn when you should begin screening and how frequently it should be done.
- If you are at high risk for breast cancer, discuss the pros and cons of taking tamoxifen with your doctor.
- Eat wisely—cut down on fats, and eat lots of fruits and vegetables; drink a minimum of alcohol; don't smoke.
- Make exercise a daily habit.

Rate Your Risk: Breast Cancer

Put a check mark after each answer. Answer all questions. Then consult the scoring key to compute your score.

Score

(+ column) (– column)

Family History

1. Have any close family members
(grandmother, mother, sister, or aunt)
been treated for breast cancer?
Yes _____ +3   No _____ 0

2. If yes, were they diagnosed before the
age of 55?
Yes _____ +2   No _____ 0

3. Have any close family members been
treated for ovarian cancer?
Yes _____ +3   No _____ 0

4. If yes, were they diagnosed before the
age of 50?
Yes _____ +3   No _____ 0

5. Have any close family members been
treated for colon cancer?
Yes _____ +2   No _____ 0

6. If yes, were they diagnosed before the
age of 50?
Yes _____ +2   No _____ 0

7. Have any close family members been
treated for uterine (endometrial) cancer?
Yes _____ +2   No _____ 0

8. Have two or more close family members _____ _____
been treated for breast cancer?
Yes _____ +3   No _____ 0

9. Have two or more close family _____ _____
members been treated for ovarian cancer?
Yes _____ +3   No _____ 0

10. Have two or more close family _____ _____
members been treated for colon cancer?
Yes _____ +3   No _____ 0

Personal History / Habits

11. How old are you?
    20–29   +1
    30–39   +2
    41–49   +3
    50 and over   +4   _____ _____

12. Are you a smoker?   _____ _____
Yes _____ +1   No _____ 0

13. How would you characterize your diet?
Low in fat to average 0
Average to high in fat +1

14. How old were you when you got
your first period?
9–11 +2   12–14 +1 points   15 or over 0   _____ _____

15. If you have experienced at least one   _____ _____
full-term pregnancy, did you first give birth:
Before age 29? –1   After age 30? +1
Not applicable 0

16. If you are past menopause, are you   _____ _____
taking hormone replacement therapy?
Yes +1   No 0

17. If yes, how long have you been

taking HRT?

Under five years   0   5–9 years   +1

10 years or more   +2

       Subtotal

       Risk Factor   +5

       (add in only if you answered

       yes to all or either #1, 3, or 8)

       Final Score

How to Score

1. Fill in the numbers in the columns at the far right.

2. Subtotal your score from the plus and minus columns.

3. Add the +5 if you answered yes to particular risk factors.

4. Compute your final score.

5. Compare your score to the Risk Factor Scoring Chart.

Breast Cancer Risk Factor Scoring Chart

   9 or below   Lowest risk

   10 to 19   Low to moderate

   20 to 29   Moderate to high

   30 or above   Highest risk

CERVICAL CANCER

ANNE IS A SINGLE MOTHER who cannot afford to be sick. But she didn't realize the chance she was taking when, as the years rolled by, she skipped her yearly visit to the gynecologist and, with it, her annual Pap test.

"I used to go every year, but then I just stopped. There was the expense, the inconvenience, and I didn't like the exam. Some of the doctors I'd had were rough and insensitive," she recalls. But two years ago, when her forty-fifth birthday arrived, Anne, conscious she was growing older, decided to put it off no longer. She'd never had any type of gynecological problem, and she was confident none would be found. So she returned home, expecting a clean bill of health. She was wrong. "The doctor called me back, and the test was abnormal," Anne said. She underwent a biopsy. Five days later, the report came back. "Precancerous cells," it read.

Anne had to undergo a surgical procedure to have the precancerous tissue removed, and she's experienced no further problems. But she still shudders when she recalls those days.

"During that time my fear was that I had terminal cancer. It was very scary. I can't help but wonder what would have happened if I hadn't had that Pap test. I don't like to think that, because I didn't have something that simple done, I might have ended up with cancer," she said.

WHAT IS CERVICAL CANCER?

Cervical cancer develops in the cervix, the part of the uterus that is connected to the upper vagina. It's the structure that widens during childbirth, enabling a baby to travel through the birth canal.

Two major types of cancer can develop in the cervix: *squamous cell cancer* and *adenocarcinoma*. Squamous cell cancers account for 85 percent of all cervical cancers; adenocarcinomas comprise the remaining 15 percent. Some think the incidences of this rarer form of cervical cancer may be gradually increasing.

Sixty years ago, cervical cancer was the deadliest cancer afflicting American women, surpassing even breast cancer. Since then both the occurrence and the death rate have plummeted. Nowadays, an estimated 13,700 cases of invasive cervical cancer are diagnosed each year, and about 4,900 women will die from it. Rates for African-American women are also declining, but if they develop it, they are twice as likely to die. This is probably because these women are more likely to be poor and less likely to get preventative health care, including Pap tests.

Since the number of women killed by cervical cancer is relatively small, why include it in this book? It's because no women should die from cervical cancer. This is a slow-growing cancer that, when diagnosed early, is highly curable. Yet, although the Pap test is effective and low in cost, many women skip getting it.

In addition, even though invasive cervical cancer is relatively rare, precancerous cervical conditions are not. In fact, they are becoming increasingly common. About 50,000 women develop these conditions, collectively known as *cervical intraepithelial neoplasia* (CIN), every year. These conditions are characterized by varying degrees of dysplasia, or abnormal tissue growth. These cellular abnormalities can range from mild to severe and progress through several stages before developing into the type of cancer that has the ability to spread. Although only a small percentage of these cases do progress into this life-threatening, invasive cancer, having a precancerous condition can lead to infertility. This is a high price to pay for a condition that is largely preventable.

"If you have a precancerous condition, you may have to invest a lot of time, money, and worry into it. Most of them can be treated without a hysterectomy, but some women do lose their ability to bear children," says Barrie Anderson, M.D., a professor of gynecology and obstetrics at the University of Iowa College of Medicine.

FACTORS THAT INCREASE YOUR RISK OF CERVICAL CANCER

Contracting a Sexually Transmitted Disease

It's not known what causes all cases of cervical cancer, but it's believed that a large proportion of them are caused by transmission of the human papilloma virus (HPV), which can manifest itself as genital warts.

Sexually transmitted diseases (STDs) are surprisingly common. Every year more than 12 million Americans contract an STD, and the problem is considered epidemic on college campuses. Human papilloma virus is one of some 20 forms of sexually transmitted diseases, which used to be lumped together under the umbrella term of *venereal disease*. But HPV is also an umbrella term; only a few strains of this virus are implicated in causing abnormalities that can lead to cervical cancer; others are linked to more harmless conditions such as genital warts. (Other serious STDs, such as gonorrhea and chlamydia, are also major causes of infertility.)

Some experts believe that all cases of cervical cancer are sexually transmitted, but not everyone agrees. There may be a small percentage of cervical cancers "that are extremely aggressive [which] may not be related to HPV or sexual activity," says Dr. John P. Curtain, an associate attending gynecological surgeon at Memorial Sloan-Kettering. Such cancers appear to follow a different course; they grow rapidly, and in their early stages they can't be detected by screening tests like the Pap smear.

Not Having Annual Pap Tests

The Pap test, known also as the Pap smear, was developed in 1943 by Dr. George N. Papanicolaou. Since then it's been credited with the 70 percent decline in the American death rate from cervical cancer. Because of the Pap smear, cervical cancer has become an unusual disease in our country, compared to countries such as Latin America, where there is little screening and cervical cancer still kills large numbers of women.

As you'll see later in this chapter, the interpretation of the Pap test is complicated, and many issues are involved in making sure yours is accurate. However, because media reports have focused on the horror stories concerning Pap tests, it's easy to get the impression that misread tests are the big problem. They're not; studies show it is *missed* Pap tests, not *misread* Pap tests, that are more likely to cost a woman her life.

In a study published in 1995 in the *American Journal of Public Health*, researchers examining the records of 428 invasive cervical cancer patients found that 29 percent of the women had never had a Pap test and another 24 percent had skipped it for at least five years. So having annual Pap tests is extremely important to conquer the odds of cervical cancer.

Becoming Sexually Active at a Young Age

Girls who begin having sex when they are teenagers may be at increased risk. When a girl reaches puberty, the cells lining her cervix undergo change, and intercourse during this period could play a role in the initiation of cervical cancer, experts believe. "The closer a woman begins sexual activity to the time she begins menstruating, the higher the overall risk is," Dr. Curtain said.

Women who have many sexual partners are also at higher risk of contracting an STD, since there is an increased probability one of those partners might have one. This is not to imply that avoiding sexually transmitted diseases is solely a woman's responsibility. She is equally at risk if she is monogamous but her partner is not, and is being exposed to HPV through his sexual activity.

As an unfortunate result of this suspected connection, many women who develop cervical cancer, or a precursor, may be treated unfairly, as Anne discovered when she went to a hospital emergency room with heavy bleeding. When the staff saw her records, she said, "I was made to feel like I must have 'done something,' or I must have had sex at an early age, or lots of partners. I was treated like I was a loose woman," Anne recalled with indignation.

Although HPV is spread conventionally through sexual contact, you can also become infected if, for example, you touch an HPV-caused wart on your partner and then touch your own genitals.

Smoking

Cervical cancer stems from cellular changes within the cervix. Smoking increases the possibility that such changes will occur. Although it's not precisely known how smoking induces such changes, it's theorized that the poisonous substances in cigarette smoke are the culprit, says Dr. Anderson.

When a smoker inhales, the toxins from the cigarette smoke enter her bloodstream. Eventually, this blood travels to the cervix. Harmless bacteria make their home in a healthy cervix. It's thought that these bacteria may interact with the toxins, transforming them into carcinogens. So, if you smoke, says Dr. Anderson, "you're bathing your cervix in carcinogens."

According to Dr. Anderson, these toxins also may damage cells in the cervix that are part of the body's immune response, which fights off potentially cancerous changes. "One doctor I know tells his patients who smoke that they are using their cervix as a toxic waste dump," Dr. Anderson adds.

Using Oral Contraceptives

Some experts say that oral contraceptives indirectly contribute to cervical cancer because women who use them may be less inclined to use condoms or diaphragms, which help protect against HPV. But there is some evidence that birth control pills directly contribute to this disease.

In 1994, *Lancet* reported that there was a higher rate of adeno-carcinoma, the rarer form of cervical cancer, among women who took oral contraceptives for more than 12 years. Those who took the pills for shorter periods had lower risk. The researchers speculated that this might be because hormones induce hyperplasia, an abnormal cellular growth in the cervix. So if you're on the Pill, an annual Pap test is a must. Also, if you've experienced any abnormal changes in your cervical tissues, you might consider changing to another form of birth control.

IF YOU'RE A DES DAUGHTER . . .

"I started feeling bad that April, but I just thought I had a recurrent yeast infection that just would not go away. I kept getting Pap smears, but they kept coming back negative. By August I was really in a lot of pain. I went to another gynecologist and she told me, straight out, "You have cervical cancer, and I need you to find out if you are a DES daughter, because if you are, then you may have other types of cancer," Sandy recalls.

Sandy was shocked. She was only 27 years old, and if she'd heard of DES, she had never given it a thought. Now it posed a threat to her life.

A synthetic form of estrogen, DES, or diethylstilbestrol, was widely prescribed for pregnant women from 1938 to 1971, when the FDA issued a warning against it. The drug, supposed to prevent miscarriages and although later found to be ineffective, was marketed under 200 brand names and was even sold as "pregnancy vitamins." The consequences for the women who took DES, and their daughters, are still with us.

Women whose mothers took DES are at increased risk for reproductive abnormalities and rare forms of cancers. One of these, clear-cell adenocarcinoma of the vagina, is very rare. It develops at much younger ages in DES daughters than in women generally, occurring between the ages of 7 and 40. Most often it is diagnosed between the ages of 15 and 22. There is no upper age limit.

Most DES daughters are now past the age when most of these

DES-related cervical cancers occur. Still, though, it is not known if they will face increased cervical cancer as they age. It's also unknown if their mothers, as they grow older, will face increased cervical cancer risk as well.

Beat Your Risk: *Ask your mother if she took DES. If so, tell your gynecologist. You will need to undergo annual pelvic exams and a certain type of Pap test. Utilize the information in the Resources section to learn more about DES so you can be certain you're getting the proper preventative care.*

HOW TO REDUCE THE RISK OF CERVICAL CANCER

Use a "Barrier" Type of Contraception

Using a condom or a diaphragm, both of which are barrier types of contraception, will protect you from sexually transmitted diseases, including HPV. Which method is preferable? A condom will help safeguard you from AIDS as well. But if you're concerned solely about cervical cancer, a diaphragm provides protection.

Unfortunately, though, most women don't take these precautions.

"It's very scary, because the women most affected are teenagers or in their early twenties who are more likely to come into contact with more partners. With young women, you are dealing with a sense of immortality. There's the typical feeling that 'nothing is going to happen to me and, if it does, I'll be so old, I won't care.' So it's very easy to get carried away and not use a condom or diaphragm," says Dr. Anderson.

Given the prevalence of sexually transmitted diseases, such forms of contraception are a must.

Beat Your Risk: Even if you're monogamous, you may be at risk if your partner has had many other partners. The adage "When you have sex with someone, you are having sex with every person that person ever had sex with" is true when it comes to HPV as well as other sexually transmitted diseases.

Don't Smoke

As noted, smoking increases the risk of cervical cancer. For more information on how to quit smoking, see chapter 15.

Eat Lots of Fruits and Vegetables

Can your choice of foods help prevent cervical cancer? The definitive answer to that question is not yet in, but research indicates that eating wisely may help.

Each of the body's cells has the ability to ward off potentially cancerous changes. Some researchers speculate that this immune response can be bolstered by vitamins, particularly vitamin A, vitamin B, folic acid (also called folate), and beta carotene. There's no evidence, though, that nutritional supplements provide the same benefits as eating foods that contain these substances. For more information on what to eat, see chapter 16.

Get an Annual Pap Test

You're probably very familiar with the Pap test, also known as a Pap smear, a simple, inexpensive test that is performed in the doctor's office. During the pelvic examination the doctor takes a sample of cells from the cervix and then sends it to a laboratory for examination.

It's important to understand that this test is not foolproof. Furthermore, there is nothing inherent in having a Pap test done that prevents cancer. It's simply a screening test—albeit an extremely important one—that allows for the detection of potential problems early on.

The Pap test is not perfect. While it is one of the best screening tests, its accuracy depends on several factors.

The major problem with the Pap test is that there is a 10 to 30 percent chance that it will falsely indicate that no cancer is present. Because of some highly publicized cases in recent years in which women who got misread Pap tests died, the quality issue has come under intense scrutiny.

Although getting a Pap test is simple, the correct reading of it is a daunting task for even the most highly trained cytologists, the test readers. Each Pap smear, it's estimated, contains about 50,000 to 300,000 epithelial cells, microorganisms, and other inflammatory material. Differentiating between normal and abnormal cells is extremely difficult. A few years ago, it was found that some labs were doing sloppy work, pressuring cytologists to work too long and process too many tests too fast. Congressional hearings were held and new regulations passed. As a result, all laboratories that handle Pap tests must now be federally certified. In addition, some laboratories may voluntarily be accredited by the College of American Pathologists and/or the Joint Commission on Accreditation of Health Care Organizations. These regulations have improved the quality of Pap test readings, but because of difficulties inherent in the test itself, there's no way of insuring that every test that is done will be perfect.

Because of this fallibility, new systems and procedures have been developed to increase the accuracy of Pap tests. One type, which goes under the commercial name of ThinPrep, processes the cellular samples differently; others use computers as a double check.

The computerized systems, Papnet and Autopap, work as a quality check by reviewing Pap test samples that have been read and classified as negative. These computers, programmed to recognize physical characteristics of abnormal cells, scan the slides, noting any samples of cells that seem to have those characteristics. The results are sent back to the cytologist for final evaluation. In 1998 the FDA approved AutoPap to automatically screen and diagnose 25 percent of the most normal Pap smears without human review. The remaining slides must be checked by humans.

The ThinPrep system processes the sample cells in a different way before they are sent to be read. In the conventional test, the cells are smeared onto a glass slide along with mucus and other cellular debris, making it more difficult to read. With ThinPrep the cells are put into a fluid that goes through a filtration process, depositing a representative layer of cells on a slide. This is designed to increase accuracy.

Whether these technologies end up being more accurate remains undetermined, notes Dorothy L. Rosenthal, M.D., director of cytopathology at Johns Hopkins University. She's concerned that the publicity surrounding these new tests has falsely raised expectations about their accuracy. These new technologies may indeed influence the practice of gynecologic cytopathology in the future, she says. But how much more accurate they are than the conventional Pap tests will not be established until additional well-controlled studies are performed. These will provide cytopathologists and medical practitioners with unbiased results on which to judge the real value of these new techniques, she wrote in an editorial published in 1998 in the *Journal of the National Cancer Institute*.

But no matter whether it's the conventional test or a newer one, the result of the Pap test is only as good as the laboratory itself. For example, in some cases a conventional Pap test that is performed and evaluated properly may be more accurate than one done by one of the newer methods if the laboratory analyzing it is not thoroughly familiar with it.

To make certain the Pap test you get is as accurate as possible, take these steps:

1. Don't douche or have intercourse during the 24 hours prior to your Pap test.

2. If possible, have the test performed in the middle of your menstrual cycle. However, it's better to have the test than to postpone it indefinitely, waiting for the perfect time.

3. Don't assume your test will be sent to a certified site for reading. Ask about it. If you want to make sure, call a nearby academic medical center or your regional office of the Health Care Financing Administration, listed with the United States Government offices in your telephone directory.

Beat Your Risk: *If you fall into a high-risk category or you have had abnormal Pap tests in the past, this elevates the level of scrutiny your future Pap tests should have. If there are questions about a Pap test you've had taken, because of excessive inflammation or blood, for example, you should have it redone.*

A Pap Test Is Not Enough

The purpose of a screening test like the Pap test is to detect a disease in its early stages, before symptoms occur. But if the Pap test is used as a diagnostic tool in a woman experiencing symptoms, the result can be tragic. The Pap test is an effective tool for detecting precancerous cells, but not for detecting cancer.

The problem is that blood and other cellular debris in the sample can mask cancer cells and hide a malignancy. Therefore a woman's test can appear normal when she actually has cervical cancer. Too often, when cancer is missed, the woman experienced symptoms, but her doctor relied on the Pap test instead of ordering a biopsy. This is especially true because cervical cancer is no longer common, and can be missed by a doctor who rarely sees a case.

If you are experiencing symptoms that may indicate cervical cancer, or any other type of gynecological cancer, make sure your doctor investigates further. Consider getting a second opinion, possibly from a gynecologist oncologist, who specializes in cancer of the reproductive tract and has more experience in detecting cervical cancer.

Pap Test FAQs (Frequently Asked Questions)

Q: How often should I get a Pap test?
A: The American Cancer Society recommends that all sexually active women, or those who have reached the age of eighteen, have an annual Pap test. However, the Society goes on to say that the test may be performed less often after a woman has had three or more negative Pap tests in a row. However, this isn't necessarily a good idea. If a woman decides to wait another year for her Pap test, she may let it slide longer. She may figure that if it's okay to skip a Pap

test, it's okay to skip her annual pelvic exam as well. This can lead to tragedy, because a pelvic exam can detect other types of cancer. In addition, since Pap tests have an estimated 10 to 30 percent rate of error, repeated testing can pick up these errors in time; an abnormality that is missed one year can be picked up the next. Another problem is that a woman may assume her partner is being faithful, but if that isn't the case, she may unknowingly become infected with a sexually transmitted disease. For all these reasons, an annual Pap test is the wisest course.

Q: Do you ever outgrow the need for Pap tests?

A: No. Almost a quarter of all cases of cervical cancer occur in women over the age of 65, and these women are most likely to die from it. Studies find that these women are lest apt to get Pap tests done, possibly because they are less likely to visit a gynecologist, which put them at risk for other gynecological cancers as well. Even if a woman is no longer sexually active, she should still maintain a relationship with a gynecologist and undergo regular Pap tests and pelvic exams.

Q: Does a woman who has undergone a hysterectomy still need a Pap test?

A: Even though you usually will not have a cervix after a hysterectomy, you still must have an annual pelvic exam. If your hysterectomy was for a cervical premalignant lesion, or cancer in any part of the uterus, you need to be checked for recurrent disease in the vagina or vulva and for ovarian cancer if your ovaries remain. Cancer of the vagina, although less common than cancer of the cervix, is also often caused by HPV, so any woman who has been sexually active needs to have a regular Pap test. Its frequency can be determined by your medical practitioner.

Q: Since lesbians don't have sex with men, do they need Pap tests?

A: Absolutely. Although women who have sex with other women are less likely to contract some types of sexually transmitted diseases, this appears not to be true for HPV. In terms of HPV, lesbians are as likely as heterosexuals to become infected. Furthermore, most lesbians have had sex with men at some point in their lives and may have contracted a virus. Even if a woman has never had sexual activity with a man, she may become infected if her partner did.

Q: If I have an abnormal Pap test, does that mean I have cervical cancer or a precursor condition?

A: No. Unfortunately, there is currently no way to determine which HPV infections will become cancerous, so they must be treated as if they all will. Chlamydia, the most common STD, and a common vaginal infection known as trichomonas can also result in abnormal Pap test results. Cervical cells sometimes can show changes during hormone treatments, including birth control pills, and revert back to normal for unknown reasons.

CERVICAL CANCER WARNING SIGNS

Early cervical cancer often has no warning signs, which is why the Pap test is so important. If you experience abnormal bleeding, this is a major warning sign that a cancer could be developing.

Abnormal bleeding is an important concept to understand. This term means:

- bleeding after intercourse
- bleeding between your periods
- bleeding if you're past menopause and not on hormones that could cause it

Basically, you should report any unexpected vaginal bleeding to your gynecologist. In cervical cancer, for example, an abrasion often forms on the cervix and begins to bleed. At first it will bleed only after intercourse or after an examination. But as the cancer progresses, it may bleed spontaneously.

Discharge from the vagina is also often noted as a warning sign of cervical cancer, but this can be misleading, because virtually all women experience discharge. However, once a cancer spreads in the cervix, it comes into contact with bacteria from the vagina, which causes it to smell foul. But most cancers are found before this happens.

Beat Your Risk: If you experience unexpected bleeding, have it checked out immediately. It could be a sign not only of cervical cancer but also of uterine or endometrial cancer.

THE BOTTOM LINE

Although rates of cervical cancer have decreased dramatically, don't be lulled into complacency; cervical cancer remains a killer. Precancerous conditions, the precursors to cervical cancer, are very curable, but treating them can be costly, worrisome, and even jeopardize your fertility. The best protection is prevention and getting any abnormal bleeding checked.

Rate Your Risk: Cervical Cancer

Put a check mark after each answer. Answer all questions. Then consult the scoring key to compute your score.

Score

(+ column) (– column)

Personal History / Habits

1. How old are you?   _____ _____
   20–39   0
   40–49   +1
   Over 50 +2

2. Are you sexually active?   _____ _____
   Yes_____ +2   No _____ 0

3. If yes, do you have sex with one partner _____ _____
   exclusively?
   Yes_____ +1   No _____ +5

4. Have you ever been treated for a   _____ _____
   sexually transmitted disease?
   Yes_____ +1   No _____ 0

5. If yes, was it caused by the human   _____ _____
   papilloma virus?
   Yes___ +3   No ___ 0   Don't know___ 1

6. Have you ever been told your Pap   _____ _____
   test was abnormal?
   Yes_____ +3   No _____ 0

7. How old were you when you got   _____ _____
   your first period?
   Under 12 _____ +2   12–14 _____ +1
   Over 15 _____ 0

8. Do you smoke?   _____ _____
   Yes_____ +2   No _____ 0

9. Did your mother take DES (a synthetic   _____   _____
   form of estrogen once widely prescribed
   for pregnant women) when she was
   pregnant with you?
   Yes_____ +3   No _____ 0
   Don't know _____ +1

10. If you practice birth control, what   _____   _____
    type do you use?
    Oral contraceptives _____ 0
    Condoms_____ –2
    Diaphragm _____ –2   Other 0
       Subtotal   _____
       Risk Factor   +5
       (add in only if you answered
       yes to all or either #5, 6, or 10)
       Final Score   _____

How to Score

1. Fill in the numbers in the columns at the far right.
2. Subtotal your score from the plus and minus columns.
3. Add the +5 if you answered yes to particular risk factors.
4. Compute your final score.
5. Compare your score to the Risk Factor Scoring Chart.

Cervical Cancer and CIN Risk Factor Scoring Chart

   4 or below   Lowest risk
   5 to 9   Low to moderate
   10 to 14   Moderate to high
   15 or above   Highest risk

7

COLON CANCER

MOST WOMEN THINK that colon cancer occurs only in men. Wrong. Colon cancer is an equal-opportunity killer, and to think that only men are vulnerable is a potentially fatal misconception. When colon cancer is detected early, there is a 70 to 80 percent cure rate, making it among the most curable forms of cancer. But once symptoms appear, the chances of a cure drop to 50 percent or even lower.

Want more proof that you should take colon cancer seriously? Here are some statistics:

• Each year, an estimated 51,200 women develop cancer of the colon, 6,800 more than men.
• Colon cancer is one of the top three cancer killers of women, along with lung cancer and breast cancer.
• Although colon cancer is seldom thought of as a women's disease, it kills 28,600 women annually, about twice the number who die from ovarian cancer.

Another myth about colon cancer is that if you develop it, you'll have to have your colon removed in an operation called a colostomy and wear a little bag for eliminating waste for the rest of your life. Because of this, people sometimes avoid getting screening tests and even ignore symptoms. But thanks to new techniques, nowadays colostomy is often not necessary.

WHAT IS COLON CANCER?

To understand colon cancer, you need to understand how your digestive system works. Its chief function is to convert food into nourishment and to store and remove waste. The large bowel, or large intestine, is the final part of the digestive tract. Tubular in shape and about five feet long, it includes the cecum, the colon, and the rectum. The cecum, which is a pouch, is the first part of the large bowel and connects the small intestine and the colon. The colon, which is the middle section of the large bowel, extends from the cecum to the rectum.

Although cancer rarely develops in the small intestine, the colon is at tremendous risk for cancer. Cells within the colon constantly grow and divide, and such uncontrolled cell growth can lead to cancer. Furthermore, the colon acts as a storage facility for food, a situation that may promote cancer.

In addition to colon cancer, cancer of the rectum should not be overlooked; an estimated 15,800 women develop it every year. Since it is sometimes difficult to ascertain exactly where a cancer has occurred, many statisticians find it easier to use the term *colorectal cancer*.

FACTORS THAT INCREASE YOUR RISK OF COLON CANCER

Growing Older

Generally, there's a 1 in 20 risk of developing colon cancer, but that risk increases with age. Only 3 percent of colon cancers arise in those younger than 40; generally, the risk of colon cancer begins to mount after the age of 55, and 80 percent of all colon cancer occurs in women over the age of 65. However, if colon cancer runs in your family, you are at risk at a much younger age.

Race

In 1973, colon cancer occurred in nearly 20 women per 100,000. By 1989, that had dropped to about 16. That drop, however, did not include African-American women, for whom the rate has stayed the same. As with other cancers, this may in part be due to the fact they are less likely to be screened for the disease. Some studies have shown that Americans of Irish, Czech, and German ancestry have a higher-than-average risk of colorectal cancer, while Mormons and Seventh Day Adventists have a lower risk; the reason for this isn't known.

Family Medical History of Colon Cancer

Knowing your family's medical history can help you determine if you may have an above-average risk for colon cancer. If you are one of the tiny percentage of women who may have inherited a rare genetic colon cancer syndrome, a genetic blood test would indeed be useful. But for most women, the non-inherited type of colon cancer poses the greater risk. In this case, your family medical history can tip you off as well.

In a study published in 1994 in the *New England Journal of Medicine*, researchers analyzed data from 87,031 women enrolled in the Nurses' Health Study. The research found that women with a family history of colon cancer were at higher risk, and the younger the woman, the higher the risk. At highest risk were women under fifty years old, especially if two or more close relatives were affected.

The risk to these women diminished as they aged, but they still remained at a slightly higher risk than women without such a family history. This emphasizes the importance of earlier colon cancer screening in women with a family history of the disease. (By the way, although this study focused on both colon and rectal cancer, the increased risk was tied only to colon cancer.)

Experts make a division between those who have a "strong" family history and those whose family history puts them at less but still higher than average risk. John Bond, M.D., chief of gastroenterology at the Minnesota Veterans Medical Center in Minneapolis, defines a strong family history as having a parent or sibling who developed colon cancer under the age of 55 or 60. If you have relatives with colon cancer clustered on one side of the family, such as aunts, uncles, cousins, or grandparents, but your mother or father never developed the disease, this translates to a family history that "is suggestive, but less strongly so," he notes.

Experts still haven't learned how strong a role heredity plays in this disease, which is also affected by such cultural factors as a high-fat diet. In this case, it seems only logical that families raised with the same habits might be at similar risk.

Inherited Colon Cancer Syndromes

In recent years several forms of inherited colorectal cancer have been identified, and genetics tests are being developed. If you believe one of these forms of colorectal cancer may run in your family, you may want to consider checking with a genetics cancer clinic.

However, it's important to recognize that our genetics knowledge is very limited. Genetic testing cannot be relied upon to uncover the majority of colon cancer cases. Although experts believe that 50 percent of all colon cancers are genetically based, the genes identified thus far probably account for only 5 percent.

That said, however, the following covers what experts currently know about the relatively rare forms of inherited colon cancer.

- *Familial adenomatous polyposis (FAP)*. The discovery of this inherited disease in 1991 paved the way for increased understanding of inherited colorectal cancer. This disease causes carpets of polyps, or growths, to appear on the colons of relatively young sufferers, and it can turn into colon cancer when they're only in their thirties. Those who inherit this rare form of colon cancer (about one in every 5,000 people) are usually aware of it, and they have their colons removed while quite young.

However, there is a second type of this syndrome known as *at-*

tenuated familial polyposis. Those with this syndrome inherit not the entire gene mutation that causes the syndrome (known as the APC gene) but only strands of it.

"If you have familial polyposis and you don't have your colon taken out, your chance of developing colon cancer is one hundred percent, whereas if you have attenuated familial polyposis, your risk is greatly increased, but it's less than one hundred percent. We don't know the number yet, but it's lower," says Dr. Scott Kuwada, assistant professor of medicine at the Huntman Cancer Institute at the University of Utah.

• *Hereditary nonpolyposis colorectal cancer (HNPCC).* This inherited colorectal cancer is divided into two types, Lynch syndromes I and II.

Lynch I: Women who inherit the Lynch I gene don't develop carpets of polyps, but they are afflicted with small numbers of them, which can progress into colorectal cancer. Lynch II: This rare disease causes not only colon cancer but also a significantly increased risk of endometrial cancer and, less commonly, ovarian cancer.

There are some other even rarer inherited types of colorectal cancer syndromes, called Gardner's syndrome, Turcot's syndrome, and Oldfield's syndrome. These cause fewer than 1 percent of all colorectal cancers.

Dr. Sidney J. Winawer, chief of gastroenterology at Memorial Sloan-Kettering, views colorectal cancer risk as a spectrum. "Familial polyposis is at the high end of the risk spectrum, but there are people who have lesser family histories, such as cancer in one or two family members, who are also at increased risk," he said.

How do you know whether you are at genetic risk for colorectal cancer? This depends in large part on knowing your family medical history. This history may warrant further investigation if:

• There is a family history of stomach, abdominal, bowel, bone, or liver cancer. In years gone by, colon cancer may have been misclassified as one of the first three types of cancer, or it may have spread to the bone or liver in later stages.
• You have relatives who developed colon cancer under the

age of 60. The younger the person at diagnosis, the stronger the chance that genetics may be playing a role.

  • There are other cancers in your family, particularly breast and/or ovarian.

Remember, though, that even if there is no colon cancer in your family, this doesn't mean you are immune. Colon cancer can occur in anyone and becomes quite common as people age.

Beat Your Risk: *One of the reasons not to be screened for the so-called breast cancer genes is that little is known about how to prevent breast cancer. This isn't the case with colon cancer. If your family history suggests that you may be genetically predisposed to this disease, you should be evaluated, preferably at a major cancer center. Then, if you learn you've inherited such a mutation, you can receive medical and psychological counseling and be given a screening test regimen. This could save your life.*

A Personal History of Colon Polyps

As you can see from the last section, the word *polyposis* figures often in terminology used to describe different types of colon cancer. Polyposis stems from the term *polyp*.

Like other tissues and organs of the body, the colon is composed of individual cells. Our cells divide as a way of repairing worn-out or injured cells. If this process goes awry, too many cells are produced. These extra, abnormal cells form harmless polyps. After a number of years, though, a polyp may turn into a malignant cancer.

Tumors that grow from the wall into the interior space of the large bowel are extremely common. Two out of every three people over the age of 65 develop them. Ten percent of these people will develop the type that can develop into cancer. Since there is no way of differentiating the type that can become malignant, the removal of these polyps is the cornerstone of preventing colon cancer.

Generally, polyps that measure one centimeter or larger are potentially dangerous and should be removed. But smaller polyps are difficult to assess. Still, if these polyps are consistently removed when they are small, the cancer is prevented.

Beat Your Risk: *The detection and removal of polyps is one of the surest ways to reduce the risk of colorectal cancer, especially in older women and women at higher-than-average risk for this disease. Usually it's the polyps that grow large and become cancerous that cause no symptoms. This is why, if you have a history of colon polyps, you must undergo regular screening tests.*

Chronic Inflammatory Bowel Disease

A history of ulcerative colitis or Crohn's disease increases your risk of colorectal cancer. These diseases cause the lining and the wall of the bowel to become inflamed. As new replacement cells are generated, the continual cell division can eventually result in cancer.

"Having inflammatory diseases of the bowel increases the risk of colon cancer. If you have multiple episodes from an early age, then the risk of colon cancer increases dramatically," notes Peter Deckers, M.D., chief of surgery at the University of Connecticut Medical School in Farmington.

If you have ulcerative colitis, your risk of developing colon cancer is estimated to be as much as 11 times higher than that of the general population. Your risk is especially high if you developed this condition as a child, you've had it for more than 10 years, and you frequently suffer attacks. Having Crohn's disease increases your risk of developing cancer in both the large and small bowel, but less so than for those who suffer from ulcerative colitis.

Remember, these cautions only apply to diseases that are categorized as inflammatory diseases of the bowel. The common stomach malady known as irritable bowel syndrome (IBS) has *not* been found to increase colon cancer risk.

A High-Fat, Low-Fiber Diet

The traditional American high-fat diet is suspected of playing a role in some forms of cancer. With colon cancer the suspected link is quite strong, and the suspected culprit is saturated fat.

Saturated fat is the substance found in butter and animal fat that solidifies when it is refrigerated. Exactly how eating a diet high in saturated fat raises the risk of colorectal cancer is not completely understood; the answer apparently lies in the way we metabolize it.

A 1990 study published in the *New England Journal of Medicine* examined the eating habits of the participants in the Nurses' Health Study. These were primarily nonvegetarians with no known major risk factors for colon cancer. The research found that the women who ate beef, pork, or lamb daily as a main meal had two and a half times the risk of developing colorectal cancer; those who ate chicken or fish instead had a lower risk. The women who ate diets high in processed meats and liver were also at increased risk. Consuming animal fats in the form of dairy products, such as whole milk, cheese, and ice cream, did not raise the risk of cancer.

The study also found that women whose diets were low in fiber had a higher risk. Eating a diet high in fiber is thought to protect from colorectal cancer because it speeds up the digestive system and spurs the elimination from our body of the animal fats we eat. Epidemiological studies, which look at the correlations between colon cancer and diet, back this up. In developing countries such as Africa, where the diet is high in fiber, the rate of colon cancer is low. Therefore, it's wise to cut down on saturated fat and increase your intake of fiber.

Fiber is not the only substance that protects against colon cancer. Although the evidence is not as strong, some studies have shown that calcium and Vitamin D are protective. Studies also have found that people who eat a lot of fruits and vegetables have a lower risk.

Because of this, researchers decided to find out if the popular antioxidants reduced the risk of colon cancer as well. But this has not been proven. In a study, reported in 1994 in the *New England Journal of Medicine*, researchers divided 864 participants (159 of whom were women) into four groups. One group was given a placebo, the other popular antioxidants (vitamins C and E and beta carotene) in differing amounts. When the patients were examined for benign tumors, which are believed to lead to colon cancer, no difference was found. This study doesn't necessarily negate the positive effects of these nutrients; the dosage may have been too small, or the vitamins may not have been taken long enough. But it seems that, at this point, taking antioxidants is not a substitute for consuming fruits and vegetables.

Beat Your Risk: *The American Cancer Society warns that eating a lot of foods that contain nitrates, such as bacon and hot dogs, when grilled, fried, or smoked, can increase the risk of not only colon cancer but also cancer of the stomach.*

Obesity

Being overweight increases the risk of colon cancer.

Smoking

Smoking is linked to colon cancer in men, and increasingly in women. Remember that women took up smoking decades later than men, and colon cancer usually afflicts older people. If you consider these two facts, it's not surprising that studies are beginning to find a link between smoking and this disease in women.

An analysis of data from the Nurses' Health Study found double the risk of colon cancer in women who had smoked for 35 years, according to research published in 1994 in the *Journal of the National Cancer Institute*. Although three and a half decades seems like a long time, it means that for a woman who took up smoking as a teenager her risk of colorectal cancer will double by the time she reaches her fifties. As the years pass, and more studies are done, the link between smoking and cancer will be strengthened, researchers expect.

OTHER POSSIBLE RISK FACTORS

The following situations may contribute, but have not been definitively linked, to colon cancer:

Having Your Gallbladder Removed

Some studies find that women, although not men, who have had their gallbladders removed may bear a slightly increased risk. However, this has not been conclusively proved.

Diabetes

Some studies show that adults who develop Type II (non-insulin dependent) diabetes may have an increased risk. However, research published in 1998 in the *American Journal of Epidemiology* reviewed the records of more than a million respondents in a cancer prevention study to learn whether diabetics were more likely to develop colon cancer. Female diabetics were found to have slightly increased risk, although less than that of male diabetics.

It's not known exactly why diabetics may have this higher risk, but one theory suggests that, because of the way their digestive system functions, their stool collects in the colon longer, possibly paving the way for cancer-causing changes. Another possibility is that the biological nutritional imbalance that raises the risk of diabetes may also do so for colon cancer.

HOW TO REDUCE THE RISK OF COLON CANCER

Cut Down on Saturated Fat, and Eat Fiber, Fruits, and Vegetables

For this form of cancer, what you eat may have a very large impact. "In fact, diet is probably the single most important thing that people can do to reduce their risk of colon cancer," says Dr. Mandel of the Minnesota Colon Cancer Central Study.

This includes eating more fruits and vegetables, which is known to reduce the risk of cancer in general. In addition, to prevent colon cancer specifically, increase the amount of fiber in your diet, and cut down on saturated fat. For more information, see chapter 16.

Exercise

Over the past twenty years, studies have found that regular exercise reduces colon cancer risk. Many of these studies were done on men, but some have also confirmed these results in women. What does exercise do? It promotes bowel movements, shortening the amount of time that potentially carcinogenic fecal material remains in the colon. This in turn may reduce cancer risk.

Don't Smoke

Smoking is linked to colon cancer risk; for more information, see chapter 15.

Screening for Colon Cancer

If the screening tests available now for colon cancer were widely employed, the death rate would drop by up to 50 percent, experts believe. This is because screening tests can detect colon polyps before they have even become cancers. This early detection is the key to curing colorectal cancer.

The importance of screening is relatively new, and many people, and their doctors, are unaware of it. So if you are at risk, even if only because you're over 50, don't sit back. Ask your doctor about screening. This is especially true for women. Research indicates that, even though screening for both men and women falls short of national goals, men are more likely to be tested. In 1997 the American Cancer Society issued updated colon cancer screening recommendations designed to encourage screening for everyone 50 years old and over. There are several screening tests, as follows:

The Digital Rectal Exam

This examination, in which a doctor inserts a gloved finger into your rectum, is the most common screening test but it picks up only 7 to 10 percent of colon cancers. Although it is still a useful test, it's more effective at detecting prostate cancer in men.

The search has been on for a better means of testing. As of now, the two most likely candidates for widespread use are the *fecal occult blood test* (FOBT) and *flexible sigmoidoscopy*.

Fecal Occult Blood Test (FOBT)

This is one of the cheapest and easiest screening tests. The FOBT does not test for cancer but for the presence of blood in the stool. You put a tiny dab of stool onto a special card for processing. When a chemical is applied to your stool, a reaction causes a change in color if blood is present. Because cancerous tumors create their own blood supply, blood in your stool may indicate the disease.

The Minnesota Colon Cancer control study ongoing at the University of Minnesota has involved 46,551 participants, divided equally between women and men. Results thus far show that annual FOBT testing cut the colon cancer death rate by 33 percent because cases were found earlier.

FOBT is not foolproof. Many noncancerous conditions, such as hemorrhoids and ulcers, also produce blood in the stool, and this test can miss a cancer because some tumors bleed intermittently, some bleed too little to be detected, and some do not bleed at all.

Flexible Sigmoidoscopy

For this test, a doctor inserts a sigmoidoscope, a lighted tubular instrument, through the anus, enabling the viewing of the walls of the rectum and the sigmoid portion of the colon, where more than half of colon cancers occur. Although a sigmoidoscopy cannot detect all colorectal cancers, it can find about 50 percent of them. A positive finding on a sigmoidoscopy is followed by a colonoscopy.

The flexible sigmoidoscopy may be skipped, and a doctor may recommend a colonoscopy directly for those at higher risk for colon cancer due to their family medical history.

Colonoscopy

Similar to a sigmoidoscopy, this procedure involves an instrument called a colonoscopy. Though a more extensive, expensive, and uncomfortable procedure than a flexible sigmoidoscopy, it is also a treatment, in addition to a diagnostic test, because the entire colon can be examined for polyps and they can be removed all at the same time.

An alternative to a colonoscopy is a *double-contrast barium enema*, which is an examination of the entire colon by means of passing a tube with barium into the intestine and taking an X ray. Because barium, a metallic chemical, is impervious to X rays, it provides an image of the intestinal tract. It should be noted, though, that while the barium enema is less expensive than a colonoscopy, it doesn't visualize abnormalities with as much clarity, and you may need to have the test redone or have a supplementary colonoscopy if the results are not clear enough.

How Often Should Screening Tests Be Done?

For Those at Average Risk

Since 70 to 80 percent of all colon cancer cases occur in adults without specific risk factors, the American Cancer Society recommends that all adults begin colon cancer screening by age 50, either with an annual FOBT and a sigmoidoscopy every five years, or by colonoscopy every ten years, or double-contrast barium enema every five to ten years. Digital rectal examination should be performed at the time of the sigmoidoscopy or the total colon examination, that is, every five to ten years. For those who undergo periodic total colon examination for screening, no annual FOBT is needed.

For Those at Moderate Risk

An estimated 15 to 20 percent of colon cancers occur in people who fall into this category. A person is considered at moderate risk if:

- They've had small polyps
- They've had one large polyp (over one centimeter) or multiple polyps of any size
- Any first-degree relative (parent or sibling) developed colon cancer under the age of 60 or two or more first-degree relatives developed it at any age
- Other relatives developed colon cancer

If you've had a single small polyp removed, you should undergo a total colon examination within three years. If that examination is normal, you can proceed with the average-risk recommendations. If you've had a large polyp, or several smaller ones removed, you should have a total colon examination within three years and then, if normal, every five years thereafter.

If you have a first-degree relative under the age of 60 who developed colon cancer, or two or more first-degree relatives who developed it at any age, you should undergo a total colon examination at the age of 40, or ten years before the youngest case in the family, whichever is earlier. This should be repeated every five years.

If colon cancer developed in any other relatives, you should discuss with your doctor undergoing average risk screening possibly before the age of 50.

For Those at High Risk

Approximately 5 to 10 percent of all colon cancer occurs in people at high risk. The first group consists of those who have been found to have one of the two hereditary syndromes, familial adenomatous polyposis (FAP) or hereditary nonpolyposis colorectal cancer syndrome (HNPCC). The other group consists of those who have one of the two inflammatory bowel diseases, ulcerative colitis or Crohn's disease.

If you suspect you have inherited one of these genetic syndromes, you should be evaluated at a specialty center, so if the mutation is confirmed, you can be put on a screening regimen. The regimen varies, depending on the type of genetic syndrome.

If you're found to carry the genetic mutation for FAP, you should begin examinations at puberty. Such persons may chose to have their colons removed or to undergo endoscopy, the examination of the colon with an instrument called an endoscope, every one to two years.

Those who are found to have inherited the HNPCC mutation should, beginning at the age of 21, undergo a colonoscopy every two years until the age of 40, and then annually.

People with ulcerative colitis or Crohn's disease also warrant special screening. Consult your doctor.

COLON CANCER WARNING SIGNS

Here are the warning signs of colon cancer:

- Changes in bowel habits, such as constipation and diarrhea
- Very dark, mahogany red, or bright red blood in or on the stool
- Abdominal discomfort
- A persistent narrowing of the stools
- The urgent, painful need to defecate
- A feeling that you cannot completely empty your bowel following bowel movements

Other symptoms may include unexplained weight loss, anemia, unusual paleness, and fatigue.

Beat Your Risk: *The stomach symptoms of colon cancer mimic that of other stomach disorders such as irritable bowel syndrome and ulcerative colitis or even the flu. It really is impossible for anyone but a doctor to make the distinction. If you don't have a chronic stomach disorder, and you are suffering such symptoms, give it several days; if your problem disappears, it was the flu. If not, see your doctor.*

THE BOTTOM LINE

If you believe you may be at risk for hereditary colon cancer, consider contacting a cancer center for a genetic evaluation. If you are over 50 or have other risk factors, ask your doctor for a screening test. Eat a low-fat diet that includes plenty of fiber. Know your own body, and if you experience any of the warning symptoms of colon cancer, see your doctor.

Rate Your Risk: Colon Cancer

Put a check mark after each answer. Answer all questions. Then consult the scoring key to compute your score.

	Score	
Family History	(+ column)	(– column)

1. Has a close relative (mother, father sister, brother, aunt, or uncle) been treated for colon cancer?
   Yes_____ +3   No _____ 0

2. Have more than one close relative been treated for colon cancer?
   Yes_____ +5   No _____ 0

3. Do you have any close relatives who were diagnosed with breast, ovarian, or uterine (endometrial) cancer?
   Yes_____ +2   No _____ 0

4. Do you have more than one close relative who was diagnosed with breast, ovarian, or uterine (endometrial) cancer?
   Yes_____ +3   No _____ 0

Personal History / Habits

5. How old are you?
   Under 50   +1
   50–64   +2
   65 or older   +3

6. Are you more than 20 pounds over your ideal weight?
   Yes_____ +2   No _____ 0

7. How would you characterize your diet?   _____ _____
   Very low fat 0
   Low to average in fat +1
   Average to high fat +2 percent
8. Do you make an effort to eat a diet   _____ _____
   which is high in fiber?
   Yes_____ −1   No _____ +2
9. Do you smoke?   _____ _____
   Yes_____ +1   No _____ 0
10. Have you ever been treated for one   _____ _____
    or more colon polyps?
    Yes_____ +3   No _____ 0
11. Do you have ulcerative colitis?   _____ _____
    Yes_____ +2   No _____ 0
         Subtotal   _____
         Risk Factor   +5
         (add in only if you answered
         yes to all or either #1, 2, or 10)
         Final Score   _____

How to Score

1. Fill in the numbers in the columns at the far right.
2. Subtotal your score from the plus and minus columns.
3. Add the +5 if you answered yes to particular risk factors.
4. Compute your final score.
5. Compare your score to the Risk Factor Scoring Chart.

Colon Cancer Risk Factor Scoring Chart

   7 or below   Lowest risk
   8 to 14   Low to moderate
   15 to 21   Moderate to high
   Above 22   Highest risk

CHAPTER 8

LUNG CANCER

CELEBRITIES FALLING VICTIM TO fatal lung cancer is not a new story, but until now they've been men, like John Wayne and Yul Brynner. Now add to the list Audrey Meadows, the woman we grew up with as Alice Kramden. Her death ushers in a grim new era for women. Inevitably, more famous female names will be added to this tragic roster. Perhaps as these deaths sadly mount, the point will be driven home that it is lung cancer that is the biggest cancer killer of women.

"Lung cancer gets lost amidst all of the attention surrounding breast cancer. It's always thought of as a man's disease. But women get lung cancer, and lung cancer is the leading cause of cancer deaths among women, higher than breast cancer," says Diane Stover, M.D., chief of pulmonary services at Memorial Sloan-Kettering.

The numbers alone are alarming. From 1960 to 1980 the rate of lung cancer doubled in men, but it leaped sixfold in women. You'd think this would merit headlines, but lung cancer seldom makes news, even though 80,100 women are diagnosed with it every year, and 67,000 women die from it. That's 23,500 more female deaths annually than from breast cancer, and those numbers are expected to rise in the coming years.

Furthermore, although we don't know why most cases of breast cancer occur, this isn't the case with lung cancer. The cause, quite simply, is smoking.

Beat Your Risk: *When discussing lung cancer, the term smoking in the past has referred to cigarette smoking. However, cigar smoking is currently gaining the favor of women as well as men. Smoking cigars also causes lung cancer.*

WHAT IS LUNG CANCER?

Lungs, which are organs composed of soft, spongy tissue, are part of the respiratory system. When we breathe, our lungs drink in oxygen, which is necessary for all the cells in our body to live. When we exhale, our lungs expel carbon dioxide, a toxic waste product of our cells.

There are several different types of lung cancer, which can develop in the lungs themselves or in the lining of the lungs. The cancer can remain confined within this area or spread cells that take root and establish themselves in distant parts of the body. Whatever route lung cancer takes, it is usually lethal.

There are basically two types of lung cancer: small cell lung cancer, which accounts for 20 to 25 percent of all lung cancer; and nonsmall cell lung cancer, accounting for 75 to 80 percent.

Small cell is the most aggressive form of lung cancer. Its small, oatlike cells occur in the tissue of the lungs, and it often is not diagnosed until it has spread elsewhere in the body.

Nonsmall cell lung cancer also has two types: squamous cell lung cancer and adenocarcinoma. Squamous cell carcinoma often begins in the large air passages of the lungs and tends to remain there for longer periods of time. Adenocarcinoma often develops along the outer edges of the lung and under the membranes of its large air passages. Squamous cell carcinoma is more common in men, and adenocarcinoma, which grows more rapidly, occurs more often in women. Adenocarcinoma often spreads through the lymph nodes, most commonly to the brain.

WOMEN, SMOKING, AND LUNG CANCER

The statistics quoted above correlate with the rate at which American women took up smoking, making it painfully obvious that smoking is responsible for the vast majority of lung cancer cases—an estimated 80 percent. The remaining 20 percent are believed to be linked to other causes, including asbestos and radon. An extremely small number of lung cancer cases have no known cause.

Can you imagine the outcry if it was learned that a single industry was responsible for almost all cases of breast cancer? But experts who deal in risk say we tend to take the dangers we become familiar with for granted. Smoking is a prime example of this.

Although lung cancer was initially thought of as a man's disease, women may be even more vulnerable to it than men. A study published in 1996 in the *Journal of the National Cancer Institute* compared male and female lung cancer patients and found the rates higher than expected in women. Differences in smoking history, baseline exposure, or body size didn't account for the difference, so it is believed that women may be more prone to damage from the toxins in cigarette smoke than men.

Three years earlier, a Canadian study published in the *American Journal of Epidemiology* found that female smokers run about twice the risk of developing lung cancer as men, and the toll may be even higher for the women who have smoked the longest and most heavily.

WHY IS LUNG CANCER SO DEADLY?

Surveys continually show that breast cancer strikes the most fear in women. But if you're stricken with breast cancer, your chances of survival are better than with lung cancer. It's also ironic that many women fear finding lumps in their breasts. A lump is an important warning sign. Lung cancer offers no such early warning signs; by the time it is diagnosed, it's often incurable.

Lung cancer may start out as a very small peripheral nodule in the lung that causes no symptoms. There's no pain, no shortness of breath, no cough. Or if it does occur in the windpipe, it may produce a cough. But many smokers mistake this for their chronic cough.

The result? By the time 80 percent of all cases of lung cancer are diagnosed, it has already advanced. When lung cancer does spread, it usually heads for other organs. In women, as noted, it especially spreads to the brain. The result is that neurological symptoms are the first sign of the disease. Initially, the diagnosis may be a brain tumor, but it's only a secondary tumor. The primary cancer is in the lungs.

Furthermore, lung cancer is very difficult to treat effectively. A small, localized tumor can be surgically removed, but lung cancer is rarely discovered this early. If the tumor has spread, radiation and chemotherapy can be used, but these methods are not very effective. Even if the tumor hasn't spread, it can still be deadly. If it develops in the lining of the lungs or the heart, it's incurable.

If lung cancer is caught before it spreads, the five-year survival rate is 49 percent. But only 15 percent of lung cancer cases are caught so early. Because of this, the five-year survival rate for lung cancer generally remains at a dismal 14 percent, close to what it was in the 1950s.

Beat Your Risk: *Lung cancer is not the only cancer that cigarette smoking causes. Cancer can develop in any of the parts of your mouth and throat that the cigarette smoke touches, including the lips, mouth, and pharynx. These cancers can, at worst, kill you and, at best, require disfiguring surgery.*

THERE'S NOT ONLY LUNG CANCER— THERE'S COPD

Smokers are at high risk not only for lung cancer but also for *chronic obstructive pulmonary disease* (COPD). Although you rarely hear of COPD, it's our country's fifth highest cause of death, and it's on the rise in women smokers. As with lung cancer, 80 percent of COPD cases are credited to smoking.

COPD is a category of diseases that includes emphysema—a disorder that damages the tiny air sacs of the lungs, making breathing difficult—and chronic bronchitis.

The damage that causes COPD begins when the smoker is young, although the disease often doesn't manifest itself for decades. "Women who get COPD usually begin smoking in their late teens. They may begin developing it in their twenties but remain unaware of it until their fifties, when they've done so much damage to their lungs that they're short of breath," says Dr. William S. Beckett, professor of environmental medicine at the University of Rochester School of Medicine and Dentistry.

Like lung cancer, COPD offers no early warning signs, so by the time breathing difficulties or shortness of breath occur, the disease is probably far advanced.

Yet this danger continues to be particularly ignored in women. "When you think 'emphysema,' you always picture a man. But women get emphysema. Women get lung disease," notes Dr. Stover.

FACTORS THAT INCREASE YOUR RISK OF LUNG CANCER

Smoking

Most cases of lung cancer are the end result of years of bathing the lungs in the carcinogens and toxic gases contained in cigarette smoke. This smoke contains thousands of chemical compounds, including some that are carcinogenic. When we breathe, our lungs retain 70 to 90 percent of these noxious compounds.

"Smoking is like taking a sticky black substance and coating the inside and outside of the lungs until all the major airways are destroyed and eventually cancer of the lung develops," Carolyn Reed, M.D., associate professor of surgery at the Medical University of South Carolina in Charleston, told the second annual Women's Health Congress in 1994.

Furthermore, these substances apparently damage DNA, the body's genetic code, paving the way for cancer. In the study done at

Johns Hopkins University, scientists analyzing patients with head or neck cancers found that smokers were twice as likely to have mutations in their p53 gene, the important tumor suppressor gene which, when improperly functioning, causes cancer.

How much do you need to smoke to develop cancer? Experts discuss this question in terms of pack years. They place at highest risk the smoker who has accumulated 20 pack years. This amount can be accrued in different ways: a person can smoke a pack a day for twenty years, two packs a day for ten years, five packs a day for four years, and so on.

But don't confuse these distinctions with real life. There's no magic number; susceptibility to cancer varies widely from person to person. Some people can smoke their entire lives and remain cancer free; for others, cancer can develop quickly.

What About "Passive" Smoking?

Smokers affect not only their own lungs, they also foul the air of others. The Environmental Protection Agency (EPA) categorizes cigarette smoke as a Class A carcinogen, along with other known cancer-causing agents such as asbestos. The EPA blames the deaths of about 3,000 nonsmokers each year on secondhand, or passive, smoke. Since lung cancer is extremely rare in nonsmokers, this figure takes on added significance.

In discussing passive smoke, two terms are used:

- Mainstream smoke, the smoke inhaled by the smoker
- Sidestream smoke, the smoke from a lit cigarette

Environmental tobacco smoke (ETS) is made up of mainstream smoke highly diluted by sidestream smoke. Researchers have concluded that ETS contains most, if not all, of the carcinogens and toxic compounds that are present in mainstream smoke. They point to studies showing that cotinine, a derivative of nicotine, can be found in the blood and urine not only of smokers but also of nonsmokers.

Studies find that nonsmokers are at low risk for lung cancer unless they're married to or living with smokers. According to a 1994 study in the *Journal of the American Medical Association*, nonsmoking wives whose husbands smoked were at a 30 percent higher risk. But a nonsmoker did not even have to live with a smoker to be at higher risk. Nonsmokers who worked with smokers were at 39 percent increased risk, and those exposed to secondhand smoke in social setting were at 50 percent increased risk. Furthermore, women raised in the homes of smokers had a lung cancer risk of nearly twice that of the women whose exposure occurred as adults.

Although a host of prestigious organizations, including the EPA, the Surgeon General, the National Research Council/National Academy of Sciences, and the International Agency for Research on Cancer, have all concluded that passive smoking increases the risk of lung cancer, many review articles in the scientific literature have concluded differently. How can this be so? While it's true that scientific studies can cause differing results, the authors of a 1998 article published in the *Journal of the American Medical Association* have a different suspicion. They reviewed 106 articles and found that the vast majority of the authors of studies disparaging the dangers of passive smoke had one thing in common—ties to the tobacco industry.

True, passive smoke can be difficult to measure, and asking people to recall the smoking behavior of those around them is very subjective. Still, the evidence indicates that it's wise not only to quit smoking yourself but to avoid being exposed to cigarette smoke in general.

For information on how to quit smoking, see chapter 15.

Family Medical History of Lung Cancer

Everyone, it seems, can point to an example of a nonsmoker who developed lung cancer and a smoker who lived into his or her eighties, nineties, or even over a hundred. Jeanne Calment, reputedly the world's oldest person, gave up cigarettes only when she reached 120, two years before she died in 1997 in France.

How can this be so? Experts have searched for an answer, and currently have settled on the explanation that the answer lies in our genes.

Lung cancer, like other cancers, is a genetic disease; it arises after certain changes have occurred in a cell's chromosomes. These changes may occur in parts of chromosomes known as genes, or they may affect an entire chromosome. The gene known as p53 appears to be defective in virtually every case of small cell lung cancer and in half the cases of nonsmall cell lung cancer. This gene usually functions as a tumor suppressor gene, one of the body's natural defenses against cancer. In its defective form, however, p53 allows lung cancer to develop, primarily when the lungs have been damaged by environmental factors such as exposure to cigarette smoke.

On the other hand, bear in mind that our genes can also protect us. So it may be a beneficial genetic factor that safeguards the lungs of some smokers from falling prey to cancer.

Although a family history of lung cancer provides the strongest link, some studies indicate that if cervical, ovarian, or endometrial cancer (also known as uterine cancer) runs in your family, this increases your lung cancer risk as well. Remember, though, smoking is a lot like playing Russian roulette, whether lung or these other cancers "run in your family" or not. If you're a smoker, there's no guarantee you won't develop lung cancer or another deadly lung disease.

A History of COPD

Having COPD, a term which encompasses emphysema and chronic bronchitis, increases your chance of developing lung cancer.

Environmental Pollutants

Although cigarette smoke accounts for the vast majority of lung cancer cases, we're also exposed to a host of other environmental pollutants, some of which are more dangerous than others. Bear in mind, though, that toxic as these gases may be, they pale in comparison to the daily assault levied by smoking.

"There are approximately a dozen occupational substances that are known to cause lung cancer. The degree of exposure to these substances isn't as well understood, but available information indicates that the risk of lung cancer from smoking overall strongly outweighs occupational and other exposures," says Dr. Beckett.

Asbestos

Probably the most familiar of these carcinogenic substances is asbestos. Asbestos is the name for a group of minerals that form as fibers and break into particles. When these particles are inhaled, lung cancer risk goes up.

Over the years the awareness of the danger posed by asbestos has grown, and we've limited our exposure. However, asbestos is still found in some materials, such as brake linings and some types of insulation. If you discover asbestos in your home, it should be left alone if it is in good condition. If it is worn or damaged, it may need to be removed. Never touch or attempt to remove asbestos yourself; hire a qualified contractor to do it. To find one, call the EPA-funded Toxic Hotline in Washington at 202-554-1404.

Since it can take twenty years for damage from inhaling asbestos to occur, even if you were exposed to particles of asbestos decades ago, you should ask your doctor about getting a chest X ray.

Beat Your Risk: *Usually, we think of asbestos as posing an occupational danger chiefly to those who work with it. But it can present a hidden danger to women who live with men who work with asbestos. They can be exposed to fibers that cling to clothing, for example, and inadvertently inhale it just by putting this clothing in the washing machine.*

Radon

A few years ago, concern about radon made headlines. Stores couldn't keep radon-testing kits in stock. Lately, this concern has diminished, as studies indicate the risk from radon may be less than originally thought.

Radon is nothing new; it's always been around—literally. A radioactive gas that occurs naturally when the uranium located in rock and soil decays, radon surrounds us. But this gas was deemed dan-

gerous when it was discovered that radon causes lung cancer in uranium workers, who inhale it in dusty, underground mines.

Obviously, since radon comes from rock and soil, we're exposed
to it outdoors, but the amount of radon is so small it poses no haz-
ard. Only when it was discovered that radon seeps into our houses in
concentrated amounts was there concern this could cause lung cancer as well. In fact, the EPA estimated that exposure could account
for 15,000 lung cancer deaths annually.

However, this figure was extrapolated using data from the uranium workers, and these miners are also exposed to silica, arsenic,
diesel exhaust, and blasting fumes. In addition, levels of radon vary
greatly from house to house. So although there is no question that
radon causes cancer in humans, it's not known exactly what threat
residential radon poses, and study findings are inconsistent.

For example, in 1994, a study published in the *New England Journal
of Medicine* branded residential radon a cause of lung cancer on a par
with that for miners. However, no such link was found in research done
in China, Finland, and Canada. Slight increases in risk were suggested
by findings in New Jersey and Stockholm. In an attempt to clarify the
issue, the authors of a 1995 article in the *Journal of the National Cancer
Institute* compared the radon exposure in lung cancer patients with that
of those who were healthy. They found no significant link.

Radon slips into homes in such ways as through cracks in floors
and walls and gaps in suspended floors, around service pipes, and in
construction joints and the water supply. To test your home for
radon, buy a home radon-test kit. If the results reveal high concentrations of radon, call in a professional radon tester to confirm the
findings. Fixing the problem involves sealing all the cracks and
openings in the foundations and then installing fans and ventilators.
In his "Home Clinic" column in the *New York Times*, writer Edward
R. Lipinski estimated the average cost of this at about $1,500. (For
more information on radon, check the Resources section.)

Air Pollution

If cigarette smoking damages your lungs, what about the toxic gases we inhale daily from car exhaust, factory smokestacks, or clouds of smog? Aren't these dangerous as well?

Those who live in polluted areas are continuously exposed to some of the same toxic gases, such as nitrogen oxide and carbon monoxide, found in cigarette smoke. They may find it difficult to breathe on days when the pollution is high.

There is evidence that this poisonous mix can damage the lungs; a study by UCLA researchers that looked at the lungs of 2,100 residents living in three heavily polluted Southern California communities found that residents there had as much respiratory damage as smokers who lived in the least polluted cities. However, whether this damage results in lung cancer and COPD isn't known.

Other Risk Factors

Tuberculosis and radiation to the chest are risk factors that increase the probability of developing lung cancer, but they affect relatively small numbers of people.

Tuberculosis (TB)

Tuberculosis, a contagious, potentially fatal infection, which can increase the risk of lung cancer due to scarring, was once a leading cause of death in the United States; it was nearly eradicated, thanks to the development of effective antibiotics. Unfortunately, though, a new epidemic of TB has sprung up, primarily in the poor sections of cities, due to overcrowding and unsanitary conditions, and because the compromised immune systems of AIDS victims makes them vulnerable to disease. This problem is especially worrisome because some strains of TB are resistant to the antibiotics used earlier.

Radiation

If you've undergone radiation to your chest for any reason, including as medical treatment for cancer, your risk of lung cancer is slightly increased. For example, survivors of Hodgkin's disease have been found to have a higher rate of lung cancer 10 to 30 years after treatment.

HOW TO REDUCE THE RISK OF LUNG CANCER

Don't Smoke

When you smoke, your lungs gradually progress through several degenerating stages of which the final one is cancer. Once you stop smoking, the cells in your lungs gradually revert to a healthier state.

But quitting smoking can be extremely difficult. That's the reason an entire section of this book, plus an extensive list of resources, is devoted to quitting smoking. This underscores the fact that, if you smoke, quitting should be your number one priority.

Eat Lots of Fruits and Vegetables

Researchers who work on lung cancer noticed that some studies found that people with this disease also happened to be those who didn't eat a lot of fruits and vegetables. Because these foods are rich in vitamin A and beta carotene, researchers decided to give these vitamins to smokers to learn if it would reduce their lung cancer risk. Thus far the answer is a discouraging no, says Curtis Mettlin, Ph.D., chief of epidemiologic research at the Rosewell Park Cancer Institute in Buffalo, New York, who has worked on these studies for years.

Two major studies—one done on Finnish men and published in 1994 in the *New England Journal of Medicine*, the other an American study that replicated it—found that not only did these supplements fail to reduce risk, they actually increased it. In fact, the American study was halted early because of this.

Dr. Mettlin still believes that the vitamins are protective. He speculates that the research failed because the participants may have been given them too late in life, or that heavy doses of supplemental beta carotene prevented other carotenoids, the other beneficial chemicals contained in produce, from being absorbed.

Although researchers still believe that these vitamins may help protect against lung cancer, apparently there are other substances in the whole foods themselves that may furnish this protection; just taking the supplements isn't enough. For more information on adding more fruits and vegetables to your diet, see chapter 16.

Screening for Lung Cancer

The screening tests outlined in this book can detect many types of diseases. But in the case of lung cancer, screening is controversial. This is because a cancer of the lung can grow for up to 10 years before it is detected by current diagnostic methods. By that time the disease is firmly entrenched, so screening is useless, many say.

Not everyone agrees. In the past, two methods have been investigated to determine if they would be useful screening tools. Here is how they stand:

Sputum Cytology

The Pap test, which transformed cervical cancer from a devastating killer into a relatively rare disease, depends on the identification of abnormal cells taken from the cervix. This test for lung cancer is similar, only it is the cells found in the sputum, or mucus that is coughed up, that are analyzed for cancer. The problem is that this method, while it is an effective diagnostic tool, does not detect cancer early enough to serve as an effective screening test for the disease.

Annual Chest X Rays

Annual chest X rays may eventually prove their worth as a screening tool for those at high risk for lung cancer, particularly smokers. Right now, though, there's a lot of controversy about them. During the 1970s, three large-scale trials, involving 30,000 men, were performed to evaluate the effectiveness of annual chest X rays and lo-sputum cytology as a screening test for lung cancer. Although the tests did detect cancer earlier, they had no impact on the death rate, says Dr. Barnett Kramer, associate director of the early detection program at the National Cancer Institute. This is because, by the time a lung cancer is big enough to show up on a chest X ray, the chance of it being cured may have already passed. The result? Although you may find lung cancer cases earlier, the victims are just as likely to die—they'll only know it longer. Indeed, no major health or cancer organization currently recommends such tests, he notes.

Case closed? Not by a long shot. Some experts retain widespread interest in the value of annual chest X rays as a screening method for detecting lung cancer. Dr. Thomas A. Sheldon, a radiation oncologist who is on the American Cancer Society's detection and treatment committee, believes that the previous research that disproved the value of chest X rays was flawed. He also contends that although these tests did not affect the ultimate mortality rate, some cancer victims may have survived longer because they received treatment earlier. Furthermore, it's not known if chest X rays would be valuable screening for women.

"Back in the 1970s, when these studies were done, there weren't as many longtime women smokers, so they were not included," Dr. Sheldon notes.

To resolve the issue, the National Cancer Institute included screening chest X rays in a study currently underway that is also evaluating screening tests for prostate, colon, and ovarian cancer. Called the PLCO study, it will include female smokers for the first time.

Beat Your Risk: *Lung cancer is a disease of former as well as current smokers. If you are a current or past smoker, ask your doctor for an annual chest X ray. Although not accepted as a widespread screening tool, this could save your life.*

LUNG CANCER WARNING SIGNS

Occasionally, lung cancer can be detected early enough to be effectively treated, even cured. So if you experience any of the following warning signs, don't ignore them:

Persistent deep, wheezing cough
Increased sputum, or mucus, which may be streaked with blood
Chronic chest pain
Belabored breathing
Recurring pneumonia or bronchitis
Difficulty swallowing
Hoarseness
Fatigue

Beat Your Risk: *Although it is not sometimes listed as a major symptom, fatigue can be a common warning sign of lung cancer. But bear in mind it is also easily overlooked or misinterpreted.*

THE BOTTOM LINE

Lung cancer is the biggest cancer killer of women, and the toll is rising. The only proven way to keep yourself from becoming a statistic is to vow to quit smoking. See chapter 15 for important information and tips.

Rate Your Risk: Lung Cancer

Put a check mark after each answer. Answer all questions. Then consult the scoring key to compute your score.

	Score	
	(+ column)	(– column)

Family History

1. Have any of your close family members _____ _____
   been treated for lung cancer?
   Yes_____ +1   No _____ 0

Personal History/Habits

2. What is your age?   _____ _____
   20–39 _____ +1
   40–49 _____ +2
   Over 50 _____ +3

3. Have you ever been a smoker?   _____ _____
   Yes_____ +4   No _____ 0

4. Do you smoke now?   _____ _____
   Yes_____ +4   No _____ 0
   (If no, skip to #7)

5. If yes, how many cigarettes do you   _____ _____
   smoke daily?
   Less than 1 pack   +1
   1 pack   +2
   1 to 1 1/2 packs   +3
   2 or more packs   +4

6. If you no longer smoke, how long ago   _____ _____
   did you quit?
   Less than 5 years ago?   –1
   6–10 years ago?   –2
   11–20 years ago?   –3
   Over 21 years ago?   –4

7. Do you live with a smoker?   _____ _____
   Yes_____ +3   No _____ 0

8. Do you work in an environment in   _____ _____
   which people smoke, such as a bar or
   restaurant?
   Yes_____ +3   No _____ 0

9. Have you ever been diagnosed with   _____ _____
   chronic bronchitis or emphysema?
   Yes_____ +2   No _____ 0

   Subtotal   _____

   Risk Factor   +5
   (add in only if you answered
   yes to #4)

   Final Score   _____

How to Score

1. Fill in the numbers in the columns at the far right.
2. Subtotal your score from the plus and minus columns.
3. Add the +5 if you answered yes to particular risk factors.
4. Compute your final score.
5. Compare your score to the Risk Factor Scoring Chart.

Lung Cancer Risk Factor Scoring Chart

  6 or below   Lowest risk
  7 to 12   Low to moderate
  13 to 18   Moderate to high
  Above 19   Highest risk

OVARIAN CANCER

IN HER MEMOIR, *It's Always Something*, the comedienne Gilda Radner writes of her tragic family history of ovarian cancer. Her aunt, cousin, and probably her grandmother all died of this disease. Yet Radner's cancer was not diagnosed until it was too late.

Ginnie is determined not to follow Gilda Radner's fate. When in her thirties she began experiencing what she called "weird gastrointestinal symptoms," her doctor assured her that they would eventually disappear. When they didn't, she persisted. Eventually, exploratory surgery revealed ovarian cancer. Since then she's researched the subject and warily monitored her own treatment. "I'm going to beat this," she says.

Every year an estimated 25,400 new cases of ovarian cancer are diagnosed, and an estimated 14,500 women die. We dread finding a lump in our breast, but that lump can be a lifesaver. Ovarian cancer offers no early warning.

The risk of developing ovarian cancer is 1 in 70, although Dr. M. Steven Piver, head of the Gilda Radner Familial Ovarian Cancer Registry at the Roswell Park Cancer Institute in Buffalo, New York, believes that based on his studies, the rate is now 1 in 55. However, since the cause of ovarian cancer isn't known, the reason for any increase isn't known either.

Although relatively rare, ovarian cancer causes more deaths than any other female reproductive tract cancer. That's because it's usually diagnosed at such a late stage. Thanks to the publicity generated by Gilda Radner's death, awareness of the disease has increased. Hopefully, as more women—and their doctors—become aware of the danger it poses, more women's lives can be saved.

WHAT IS OVARIAN CANCER?

Ovarian cancer develops in the ovaries, the two female reproductive organs that produce egg cells, or ova. An ovary can balloon to the size of a grapefruit without providing any hint that something is amiss.

When ovarian cancer is detected at an early stage, there is an 85 percent chance of surviving for five years or more. But it's usually not found that early. Seventy percent of the time, the cancer already has spread beyond the pelvic region.

Ovarian cancer poses a problem for doctors, who in medical school learn the adage: "When you hear hoofbeats, look for a horse, not a zebra." That's their way of saying that common symptoms are almost invariably due to common maladies. Since ovarian cancer is a rare disease with symptoms that mimic everything from flu to infection, it's often overlooked.

OVARIAN CANCER RISK FACTORS

The vast majority of ovarian cancer cases—an estimated 95 percent—occur in women without known risk factors. The exception is having close relatives who developed the disease. Other possible risk factors only slightly increase risk.

FACTORS THAT INCREASE YOUR RISK OF OVARIAN CANCER

Growing Older

Ovarian cancer occurs most often in women who are 55 to 69 years old, and the rate declines slightly after the age of 80. But younger women can develop ovarian cancer.

Beat Your Risk: Too often, when a disease becomes known as occurring more often in older women, that is misinterpreted to mean it never occurs in younger women. If a doctor tells you this, be skeptical. If treatment doesn't help, and your symptoms persist, make certain your concerns are addressed.

Race

Although African-American women face higher rates for many of the diseases in this book, this is not true for ovarian cancer. In this case white women are two-thirds more likely to develop ovarian cancer. The disease is very rare in Asian women; in contrast, Jewish women have a slightly higher rate than average.

Family Medical History of Ovarian Cancer

As with breast cancer, many women erroneously believe that if there is any ovarian cancer in their family at all, they are doomed to develop it. This is false. Only the tiniest fraction of this group, those with multiple relatives with the disease, fall into that category. Having one close relative, even a mother or sister, raises the odds by only 5 percent. If you have two close relatives, that figure rises to 7 percent. However, within this group of women with that 7 percent risk is a critically important subgroup of 3 percent who have a 50 percent chance of having inherited the genetic mutation that causes ovarian cancer. They are at the highest risk.

There are three types of these inherited ovarian cancer syndromes, as follows:

- *Site-specific ovarian cancer syndrome.* This type, which involves only ovarian cancer, is indicated by two or more first- or second-degree relatives with the disease.
- *Breast-Ovarian cancer syndrome.* This type of cancer is caused by the genetic mutation BRCA1, which is known as the breast cancer gene; it raises the risk for ovarian cancer as well. It may be indicated by families in which there are multiple cases of both breast and ovarian cancer.
- *Hereditary nonpolyposis colorectal cancer* (known also as Lynch II syndrome). Women who inherit this genetic condition may develop ovarian cancer, although the risk of endometrial cancer is higher. Stomach and renal cancer can also be seen in some families.

Is There Ovarian Cancer in Your Family?

Here are the clues that might suggest you come from a family with inherited ovarian cancer.

1. *You have more than one close relative with it.* According to Dr. Piver, ovarian cancer occurs in women with two or more first-degree relatives who have the disease. They are usually mother and daughter, or two sisters. Furthermore, almost half of these families reported having three or more relatives with ovarian cancer. Women who had only second-degree relatives with breast cancer, such as aunts or grandmothers, were also at an increased, but lesser, risk.

2. *Your relatives developed ovarian cancer at a younger age than most other women.* In Dr. Piver's study, the average age of the mothers was 59 and of the daughters 48. Most women who develop noninherited ovarian cancer are in their sixties.

Determining if there is ovarian cancer in your family can be a challenge. When Gilda Radner was first diagnosed, she believed that only one person in her family had been afflicted. But upon investigating, she found her family was riddled with it.

Radner's experience shows that memories can be faulty and family medical history fuzzy. Deaths recalled as "abdominal cancer" or "stomach cancer" may actually have been ovarian. Cancers remembered as breast cancer may have originated in the ovary and spread to the breast. Checking hospital records and/or death certificates can provide this information.

A Genetic Connection

Breast cancer victims are more likely to develop ovarian cancer. Likewise, women with ovarian cancer have a heightened risk of breast cancer. This is the case no matter whether the original cancer was inherited or not. As noted earlier, the defective gene, BRCA1, may cause breast cancer, ovarian cancer, or both.

But not everything is known about this gene. For instance, it's been found that a woman who inherits this genetic mutation has a higher risk of developing breast cancer than ovarian cancer. Why is that so? The answer is not yet known. One theory is that this genetic mutation may also play a role in the development of common forms of breast and ovarian cancer that are, as yet, not considered inherited.

Beat Your Risk: *The genes for the known inherited ovarian cancer syndromes discussed in this chapter can be passed down through either your father's or your mother's side of the family. Because these are "female" cancers, don't assume they can be passed down by only female relatives. Check the paternal side of your family tree as well.*

Certain Hormonal Factors

Advancing age and your family's medical history are the strongest risk factors for ovarian cancer. But there are some factors that, to a lesser degree, may influence your risk. The risk of developing ovarian cancer is apparently influenced by hormonal changes and other factors that are related to the reproductive system—the menstrual cycle and a woman's fertility. If you're infertile, you've never been pregnant, or if you've given birth to your first child after the age of 35, your risk of developing ovarian cancer is slightly higher.

Doctors aren't certain exactly what accounts for the increased risk, but there are several theories. First, the more times a woman ovulates over the course of her life, the higher her risk for ovarian cancer is believed to be. Every month a woman releases an egg, which bursts through a follicle sac from her ovary. This tear is repaired through the mechanism of cell division. With cell division comes the potential for a cancer-causing genetic mutation. When a woman becomes pregnant, her body gets a nine-month rest from this continuous cycle. Less mutations may equal less risk.

Bolstering this theory are studies which show which, for each child a woman has, her ovarian cancer risk diminishes. Even women whose pregnancies end in miscarriage or stillbirth have a lesser risk, according to some studies.

On the other hand, women who fail to become pregnant, despite long periods of unprotected sex, or women who have been treated unsuccessfully for infertility, are at slightly higher risk. The speculation here is that these women may have an ovarian disorder that both prevents pregnancy and may lead to cancer.

Other Possible Risk Factors

Some other factors may raise your odds, although the strength of their impact is controversial.

Infertility Drugs

An increasing number of infertile women have developed ovarian cancer over the years. Some of these women have taken infertility drugs, but it's not known if these medications are to blame for the increase. A 1992 study in the American Journal of Epidemiology found that women who underwent treatments with the three most popular fertility drugs—clomiphene, Pergonal, and hCG (human chorionic gonadotropin and urofollitropin)—did appear to have a slightly increased risk. Two years later a study in the same journal, using a larger number of women, found that those who took the most popular fertility drug on the market, clomiphene, for over a year doubled their risk of ovarian cancer. Since ovarian cancer is rare, the number of women who developed the disease was 11, but this was nearly three times the expected number of cases. But other studies, including more recent ones, have found no increased risk at all.

If there actually is an increased risk, the reason isn't known, but it's theorized that since these drugs increase ovulation, there are more ovary ruptures resulting in more repairs, and more possibilities for cancer-inducing cellular mutations. However, even if there is an increased risk, the number of women who develop ovarian cancer is very small, and becoming pregnant may provide protection against ovarian cancer and mitigate this added risk.

Eating a High-Fat Diet

No one knows for certain what causes ovarian cancer, but the same arguments against eating a high-fat diet to help prevent breast cancer are echoed by those working to find ways to reduce ovarian cancer risk. As with breast cancer, Japanese women, who eat a low-fat diet, have a low rate of ovarian cancer, notes Dr. Piver. Although this contention is far from certain, there are a few studies to back it up. A Canadian study, published in 1994 in the *Journal of the National Cancer Institute*, compared 450 Canadian women with newly diagnosed ovarian cancer with 540 healthy women. The researchers found that for each additional 10 grams of saturated fat consumed, the odds of ovarian cancer increased by 20 percent. An earlier study, published in 1990 in the *American Journal of Epidemiology*, found that whole-milk drinkers were at higher risk than low-fat milk drinkers, although the researchers acknowledged they couldn't tell whether this was due to the dairy sugar in the milk or if women who use low-fat milk eat a lower-fat diet in general.

Hormone Replacement Therapy

Researchers speculate that the use of postmenopausal estrogen could increase the risk of ovarian cancer by promoting the overgrowth of cells in the ovary, which may then result in cancer. This theory is similar to the theory that hormone replacement causes breast cancer, but with ovarian cancer the link is much more tenuous because research findings are contradictory. For more information, see chapter 18.

Beat Your Risk: *Talcum powder, deodorizing body powder, and deodorizing spray, when used on the genitals, are linked to ovarian cancer, some studies find. Chemically, talc is related to asbestos, and it's theorized that particles may migrate from the vaginal area into the pelvic cavity, and indeed such particles have been found within ovarian tissue. The reason for the effect of the other substances is not known, but there may be chemical similarities. So play it safe, and don't use them on your genitals or on sanitary napkins.*

What about Ovarian Cysts?

Ovarian cancer is rare, while ovarian cysts—abnormal, fluid-filled swellings in the ovary—are common. Ovarian cysts are benign in about 95 percent of the cases, and usually disappear without treatment.

Having an ovarian cyst does not raise your risk of ovarian cancer. However, in very rare cases they can become cancerous. They can also become painful, so if a cyst doesn't disappear by itself, it may need to be surgically removed. Usually the ovary is left intact, except in cases where the cyst is too large to make that possible. Since having ovarian cysts doesn't increase the risk of ovarian cancer, no special monitoring or screening is required.

Beat Your Risk: *If you develop an ovarian cyst, your doctor may advise you to do nothing, and wait to see if it shrinks of its own accord and vanishes. On the other hand, if the cyst continues to grow, or causes symptoms, have it evaluated further and possibly surgically removed.*

HOW TO REDUCE THE RISK OF OVARIAN CANCER

For women who are at average but no particular added risk of ovarian cancer, there are no preventative measures known at the moment, other than following general cancer-preventative guidelines such as eating lots of fruits and vegetables, cutting down on dietary fat, and having an annual pelvic exam. The following measures are for women at higher-than-average risk.

Consider Using Oral Contraceptives

Although millions of women use oral contraceptives, most news coverage about them has focused on adverse side effects, not potentially beneficial ones. So most women are unaware that oral contraceptives don't increase the risk of ovarian cancer; on the contrary, they may decrease it.

For example, a 1994 study reported in the journal *Obstetrics and Gynecology* found that women who were at higher-than-average risk for ovarian cancer because they'd never given birth could bring their risk down to average by using birth control pills for five years. Furthermore, women with a family history of ovarian cancer brought their level even below average by taking birth control pills for over 10 years.

Does this mean you should take birth control pills solely to reduce your risk of ovarian cancer? Not necessarily. For one thing, this study didn't determine whether oral contraceptives prevent ovarian cancer or simply postpone it until later in life. Also, the study reviewed only the effect of the pill on ovarian cancer, not on other health risks that oral contraceptives may increase.

On the other hand, the study demonstrates the need for more research to determine if oral contraceptives could be a valuable ovarian cancer preventative for women who are at increased risk. Currently women who take the Pill are encouraged to go on "Pill vacations," but this could blunt the apparent preventative effect.

Consider Tubal Ligation

If you've undergone sterilization by tubal ligation (commonly known as "having your tubes tied"), your odds of developing ovarian cancer are just two-thirds that of other women, according to the Nurses' Health Study, published in 1993, in which 121,700 nurses participated. Furthermore, women whose uteruses were removed, but not their ovaries, had a slightly lower risk of ovarian cancer, although not as low as the women who had their tubes tied.

The reason is not known, but one theory is that women who have had their tubes tied sometimes ovulate less often, which can translate into reduced ovarian cancer risk. Alternatively, there may be some other beneficial effect on hormone levels not yet known.

Preventative Removal of the Ovaries

When Ceil is asked her age, she answers fifty with a note of surprise in her voice. "I never thought I'd live until my fiftieth birthday," she says.

"I remember standing in the cemetery with my father when I was twenty, looking down at the grave of the aunt I had been named for. I asked my father what she died of. He looked around to make sure that no one was listening and then whispered, 'Ovarian cancer.'" Eventually Ceil learned her father's mother had also died of ovarian cancer. A few years later, a cousin on her father's side of the family died of the disease as well. At that time, Ceil recalls, "I went into shock."

Ceil began considering having her ovaries removed, but in those days, she recalls, doctors refused to discuss it. But when she was 44, she went to a gynecologist who, instead of arguing, agreed with her. Immediately after the operation, Ceil felt her death sentence was lifted. Since her surgery still another cousin on her father's side of the family has developed the disease.

Prophylactic oophorectomy, the preventive removal of the ovaries in women at high risk for ovarian cancer, is performed at about age 35, or when childbearing is completed. It is at this age that the threat of ovarian cancer begins to mount.

But it remains a controversial practice. Among the advocates is Dr. Piver, who argues, in a 1995 issue of the *Journal of Women's Health*, that the surgery could save as many as 3,200 women every year. Not everyone agrees. In the same issue, Dr. William T. Creasemen of the Medical University of South Carolina in Charleston, disagrees and calls for the use of birth control pills and tubal ligation to reduce the risk instead.

Bear in mind, though, that even the removal of the ovaries does not completely eliminate the possibility of cancer. A related type of cancer, *primary peritoneal carcinoma*, can, on rare occasions, still occur within the pelvic region.

If your family medical history indicates you may be at increased risk, you can receive the information you need to make decisions by having an evaluation at a specialized cancer center. Eventually, genetic testing may provide a more definitive answer for women who want to know if they should have their ovaries removed because it will tell them if they've inherited the genetic mutation that may cause it. But right now the same arguments against genetic testing for breast cancer, including the problems of accuracy, confidentiality, and potential discrimination, apply to ovarian cancer.

Screening for Ovarian Cancer

With a disease as insidious and deadly as ovarian cancer, it would seem logical that all women should be screened for it. Unfortunately, the quest for a suitable test has thus far proved elusive.

To be considered for use as a screening tool, a test must be cost-effective, proven to save lives, and pinpoint the disease with reasonable accuracy. In 1994 the National Institutes of Health convened a blue-ribbon panel to study all the currently available screening methods. The panel reluctantly concluded that no such acceptable screening tool yet exists.

The problem is that those available, which are valuable for diagnosis and to monitor treatment, are unsuitable for screening because they result too often in false positives: they may report cancer where none is present. This can result in unnecessary exploratory surgery. For these women, who make up the majority of those tested, "the risk may outweigh the benefits," the panel concluded. The National Institutes of Health did, however, recommend that *all* women have their comprehensive family history taken by a doctor who is knowledgeable about the risk factors associated with ovarian cancer, and undergo an annual pelvic examination as part of their routine medical care. If women who are not at particularly high risk still wish to be screened, they are encouraged to do so as part of research trials. Just such a trial, the PLCO (Prostate, Lung, Colorectal, and Ovarian Cancer) screening trial, is currently underway. It will seek to find out if screening is useful for older women whose age puts them at increased risk for ovarian cancer. For information on this test, or other research trials, call the National Institutes of Health at 1-800-4-CANCER.

Here's a rundown on the tests that can detect ovarian cancer and their pros and cons when used for screening.

Pelvic Exam

This is not, of course, a test only for women at increased risk for ovarian cancer. All women should have annual pelvic exams. The problem with using only a pelvic exam to detect ovarian cancer is that once a tumor grows large enough to be felt, it is very likely to be at a late stage.

Transvaginal Ultrasound

This diagnostic test involves inserting a wandlike probe inside the vagina to measure sound waves and create a picture of the internal organs. Although this technique can find growths, it cannot distinguish whether they are malignant or benign. To enhance it, a technique known as color-flow Doppler is added. This tool, similar to what is used on the weather maps on television, is used to detect whether a suspicious mass has its own blood supply; if so, it may mean it is malignant. A variety of other imaging techniques are also being experimented with, including MRIs and PET scans.

The CA 125 Test (and Other Similar Blood Markers)

After the death of Gilda Radner, a publicity campaign was mounted urging women to undergo CA 125 testing, a type of blood test that can uncover early ovarian cancer. Recently another marker, CA 125-II has been developed; its readings have less day-to-day variation. CA 125 stands for cancer antigen 125, a blood protein that is produced by ovarian tumors; an estimated 90 percent of ovarian tumors produce this antigen.

CA 125 and CA 125-II tests are done to monitor the success of ovarian cancer treatment, but they aren't accurate enough to detect tumors. Endometriosis and other benign conditions can generate their antigen, or the level can be elevated for no known reason. So using these tests for screening can result in false positives, undue alarm, and unnecessary surgery. And in early stages of ovarian cancer, the antigen may not be present, leading to a potentially tragic sense of false security. Hopefully, more accurate blood-marker tests will eventually be developed as a screening tool.

Screening for Women at High Risk

If you are at higher-than-average risk for ovarian cancer because of your family history, especially if you have two or more first-degree relatives with ovarian cancer, you should begin screening by the age of 25.

Such a regimen may include semiannual pelvic examinations, transvaginal pelvic ultrasound testing, and the CA 125 blood test. Long-term studies are still needed to confirm whether such screening is effective, but this is currently the best procedure available.

If you have one close relative with ovarian cancer, or have other reasons to believe you may be at increased risk, contact an ovarian cancer screening clinic to learn if screening is appropriate for you (see the Resources section).

OVARIAN CANCER WARNING SIGNS

Although little is currently known about how to prevent ovarian cancer, there are ways to reduce your risk of dying from this dread disease. The cornerstone is recognizing warning signs. As you'll see, this is often not an easy task.

The warning signs are:

Menstrual disorders (abnormal bleeding and postmenopausal bleeding)
Abdominal swelling, bloating
Indigestion
Vague but persistent stomach complaints
Frequent urination
Constipation

This list of symptoms is pretty vague, and that's the problem. It's unknown if Gilda Radner could have been saved had her cancer been diagnosed when she first sought help for her symptoms of pain, bloating, and fatigue, but she could have at least lived longer had her cancer been found earlier, according to Dr. Piver. But months dragged on while Radner went from one misdiagnosis to another.

Beat Your Risk: *Although this is not commonly listed as a warning sign, women with undiagnosed ovarian cancer often complain of a sense of abdominal fullness, even when they should be hungry. This can be due to a fluid buildup because of the cancer. This symptom is often misdiagnosed as a hiatal hernia or gallbladder disease.*

To the parents of Julie, who died at the age of 29 of ovarian cancer, Gilda Radner's story is only too familiar. When Julie first became ill, her parents recall, she complained of back pain and nausea, and even though she had little appetite, she seemed to be gaining weight. She was extremely tired, and later on she ran a fever. She was offered a variety of explanations. "One doctor told her it was PMS, another told her it was pelvic inflammatory disease, another said endometriosis. No one ever mentioned cancer," recalls Jack, her father. This went on for several months. Julie was given vitamins and antibiotics, all to no avail. She did undergo an ultrasound, and even though the results were suspicious, they were brushed aside. Finally, after exploratory surgery, advanced ovarian cancer was found.

In Julie's case, her parents believe, her youth blinded her doctors. "They kept saying she was too young to have cancer," said her father.

Julie's story sounds tragically familiar to Ginnie, who was diagnosed with ovarian cancer at the age of 36. "I go back to my journals and I read that I felt horrible. I was tired, I was bloated, I felt disgusting. And I had vague pain. I have endometriosis, so I'm accustomed to vague abdominal pain, but this was different. I had a lot of weird gastrointestinal symptoms. Every three weeks I'd run a low-grade fever and get diarrhea, gas, and bloating," she recalls.

Because of the vagueness of its symptoms, it seems understandable that ovarian cancer is so often overlooked. But Dr. Ellika Andolf takes issue with this. In a 1993 article in the journal *Clinical Obstetrics and Gynecology*, Dr. Andolf noted that out of 172 women with ovarian cancer, more than half had reported symptoms. But the majority complained of stomach problems and were not tested for ovarian cancer. Only a tiny minority—12 percent—experienced vaginal discharge or bleeding, and only these were properly tested. This demonstrates that if a woman experiences stomach complaints for no explicable reason, she should be tested for ovarian cancer, Dr. Andolf contends.

For Ginnie, the bottom line is that women need to be aware of how they normally feel and be assertive in getting help if they recognize something is wrong. "Many women are very aware of how they look and what they weigh, but they don't concentrate on how their body should feel," she said.

Beat Your Risk: *If you are at higher-than-average risk for ovarian cancer, have been told your symptoms are due to an ovarian cyst but they don't go away, or have other reason to be concerned, consider seeing a gynecological oncologist—a gynecologist who specializes in cancer. Many gynecologists see only a few cases of ovarian cancer in their entire career, if that, so they may not be as skilled in diagnosing it.*

THE BOTTOM LINE

Ovarian cancer is very rare, but it's deadly. To help guard against it, become aware of your body. Know what is normal for you and what isn't. Get annual pelvic exams, learn your family's medical history, and, if you are at higher-than-average risk for ovarian cancer, get evaluated at an ovarian cancer early detection program.

Rate Your Risk: Ovarian Cancer

Put a check mark after each answer. Answer all questions. Then consult the scoring key to compute your score.

	Score	
Family History	(+ column)	(– column)

1. Do you have any close relatives _____ _____
   (grandmother, mother, aunt, sister) who
   have been treated for ovarian cancer?
   Yes_____ +3   No _____ 0
2. Has a second close relative been treated _____ _____
   for ovarian cancer?
   Yes_____ +3   No _____ 0
3. Have any close relatives been treated _____ _____
   for breast cancer?
   Yes_____ +3   No _____ 0
4. Have any close relatives been treated _____ _____
   for both breast and ovarian cancer?
   Yes_____ +3   No _____ 0
5. Have any close relatives been treated _____ _____
   for colon or uterine (endometrial) cancer?
   Yes_____ +3   No _____ 0

Personal History/Habits

6. What is your age? _____ _____
   Under 35   0
   35–54   +1
   54–59   +2
   Over 60   +1
7. How old were you when you got your _____ _____
   first period?
   9–11   +3
   12–14   +2
   15 or over   0

8. How old were you when you reached
   menopause (add one year to your age
   when you had your final period)?
   Under 45   +1
   45–52   +2
   53 or over   +3
9. Are you infertile?
   Yes_____ +2   No _____ 0
10. Have you ever taken infertility drugs?
    Yes_____ +2   No _____ 0
11. Have you taken oral contraceptives
    for 10 years or more?
    Yes_____ –2   No _____ 0
        Subtotal
        Risk Factor   +5
        (add in only if you answered
        yes to all or either #1, 2, or 4)
        Final Score

How to Score

1. Fill in the numbers in the columns at the far right.
2. Subtotal your score from the plus and minus columns.
3. Add the +5 if you answered yes to particular risk factors.
4. Compute your final score.
5. Compare your score to the Risk Factor Scoring Chart.

Ovarian Cancer Risk Factor Scoring Chart

6 or below   Lowest risk
7 to 13   Low to moderate
14 to 20   Moderate to high
Above 21   Highest risk

CHAPTER 10

SKIN CANCER

A LL THE SEATS in the large waiting room were filled with people who had come for free skin cancer screening, a testament to the growing awareness of the dangers of this disease. Among the early arrivals to the clinic was Valerie, with her 11-year-old daughter, Teresa, in tow. They come every year.

"My mother, my father, and my two sisters have all had skin cancer in different forms. My mother has had skin grafted from her legs to her face. My father has had less serious bouts," said Valerie, who is 41.

Generally, skin cancer, although it can be disfiguring, is a less serious form of cancer. But melanoma, which forms a small percentage of skin cancer cases, is one of the most deadly forms of cancer. And the incidence of both skin cancer and melanoma is rising.

WHAT IS SKIN CANCER?

Approximately one million cases of highly curable forms of skin cancer are diagnosed every year. The most serious form of skin cancer, melanoma, is diagnosed in about 41,600 persons annually.

However, Dr. David J. Leftell, chief, section of Dermatologic Surgery Unit at the Yale University School of Medicine, points out that when diagnosed early, melanoma has a high cure rate.

Melanoma kills approximately 7,300 people annually, one-third of them women. But even the less serious forms of skin cancer can result in costly, traumatic, and disfiguring surgery.

This is a mounting problem because all forms of skin cancer rates are rising more quickly than expected. In 1981 experts created a computer model to measure melanoma risk in the United States. Back then they estimated that 1 in 250 Americans would develop melanoma, a number which would rise to 1 in 150 by 1999. That number was reached in 1985 and has been surpassed. At the current pace, the rate will climb to 1 in 75 Americans by the year 2000, according to Darrell S. Rigel, M.D., writing in 1996 in the journal *CA: A Journal for Cancer Clinicians*.

More men than women die of melanoma, possibly because women are more careful about checking their bodies and are able to catch abnormalities in time for treatment. But when a woman in her late twenties develops skin cancer, it's most often melanoma.

Skin cancer develops from uncontrolled cellular growth, in a way similar to the way cancer develops in other parts of our bodies. Every day old skin cells die and slough off, to be replaced by new ones. If this orderly pattern of cell division becomes uncontrolled, skin cancer is the result.

The Three Types of Skin Cancer

Our skin is actually our body's largest organ. The skin is made up of two main layers, the (outer) epidermis and the (inner) dermis. The epidermis is made up of three cellular layers. The outermost layer is flat, scalelike cells called *squamous cells*; the middle layer consists of round *basal cells*; buried beneath that is a layer of cells known as *melanocytes*, which produce the pigment called *melanin*.

Just as there are three layers of skin, there are three different kinds of skin cancer: *basal cell*, *squamous cell*, and *melanoma*. Both basal cell and squamous cell carcinoma arise from the most common skin cells, those that are closer to the surface. Melanomas, on the other hand, arise from the melanocytes, the cells that produce melanin.

Conquer the Odds: *Although some types of skin cancer can grow and must be removed, they don't normally have the ability to spread to other organs of the body. Melanoma does have the ability to spread, which is what makes it so deadly. This is why skin cancer must be detected early.*

Basal Cell Carcinoma

This most common form of skin cancer accounts for about 80 percent of all cases. It usually affects people over the age of 45, and for unknown reasons men have twice the risk that women do. This cancer affects people all over the United States, but those in sunnier regions are more at risk; the biggest cause appears to be sun exposure.

Basal cell carcinoma is a slow-growing cancer that rarely spreads to other parts of the body, but if left untreated, it can invade and destroy nearby bone and cartilage.

Although most basal cell carcinomas occur in older men, there is one type that may occur more in younger women. This type, called the *morpheaform* basal cell carcinoma, or aggressive-growth basal cell cancer, can appear similar to a flat, yellowish or whitish scar. Sometimes people with this type notice a "scar" but cannot remember an incident in which they were injured. This form of skin cancer is problematic because it is like an iceberg: the majority of the cancer lurks beneath the surface. In a study conducted by Dr. Leftell, he found it to be more common in women under the age of 35.

Squamous Cell Carcinoma

The second most common type of skin cancer, squamous cell, strikes at least 100,000 Americans every year, killing 2,000. This faster-growing type of cancer can sometimes spread to other organs. Even though this occurs in only 2 percent of the cases, the figure rises to 20 percent for cancers on the lips or when developing in scars from burns or X rays. So unless it is treated early, squamous cell carcinoma can be quite serious.

This cancer more often occurs in men, possibly because they work outdoors more often. Sun exposure appears to be the biggest cause. Other possible causes include chronic ulcers, burns, and prolonged contact with certain industrial chemicals. People who undergo immunosuppressive therapy following organ transplantation or during other illnesses are also prone to this cancer, as well as to basal cell carcinoma. Apparently this therapy impairs the body's ability to fight the growth of these skin tumors.

Together, basal and squamous cell cancers are known as *nonmelanoma* skin cancers, to distinguish them from melanoma.

Melanoma

Known more ominously as *malignant melanoma*, this cancer begins in the skin, often in a mole already present or in one that appears suddenly. This insidious form of cancer can grow quickly and, although appearing quite small, spread to other organs. The five-year survival rate for melanoma, when found before it has spread, is 95 percent, but the rate is only 16 percent if it has spread to other organs in the body. For this reason early detection of melanoma is vitally important.

If you want to know how dangerous melanoma can be, ask Carol, 42, the mother of two daughters, who has been battling melanoma for four years.

"I thought I had no risk factors for melanoma in my family, but I was born with a lot of moles. There was a large, two-tone one on my back, and when it started to itch, I knew something was wrong. The mole was biopsied, and that's when I discovered that I had melanoma. By then it had spread to my groin," she said. She underwent surgery, but after a year the melanoma had spread to her left breast. She underwent a mastectomy and is currently in remission.

Superficial spreading melanoma accounts for 70 percent of the cases. It occurs more commonly in women and can develop from a preexisting mole. It can arise anywhere but usually appears on the lower legs or upper back.

Nodular melanoma is a rare, fast-spreading melanoma that usually occurs in men. The moles appear suddenly and may resemble blood blisters, although they may range in color from blue-black to white.

Lentigo maligna melanoma occurs most often in people over 50; these moles usually appear on the face, ears, neck, or other parts of the body that have been exposed to the sun for years.

Acral lentiginous melanoma usually occurs in African-Americans and Asians. This particularly deadly form often has bluish black or brownish black moles that are flat with bumpy areas.

FACTORS THAT INCREASE YOUR RISK OF SKIN CANCER

Growing Older

Since it takes decades for sun damage to skin to accumulate, skin cancer is most likely to occur in women over 40. But cases of skin cancer are being seen in younger and younger women. "My colleagues in California are seeing an increased incidence of skin cancer in girls in their late teens. Even here on the East Coast, I've had patients in their early twenties, which you never would have seen in the past," Dr. Leftell says.

He believes this is due to changes in lifestyle, as young people spend more time in the sun than previous generations. This is true despite the emphasis on using sunscreen, which is relatively recent and has limitations, as you'll see.

Race

Eighty percent of skin cancer and melanoma cases occur in whites, as compared to blacks or darker-skinned minorities. In contrast, melanoma occurs in blacks extremely rarely. This does not, however, mean that blacks are immune. They are vulnerable to a rare form of melanoma that is believed to be inherited and that occurs in the areas of lighter skin not usually exposed to the sun, such as the palms of the hands, the soles of the feet, under the fingernails, and in the mouth.

Beat Your Risk: *If you're a light-skinned Latina or a member of another lighter-skinned minority group, you are vulnerable to skin cancer. It's the color of the skin that makes the difference, not your surname.*

Family Medical History of Skin Cancer and Melanoma

Like other cancers, skin cancer is influenced by genetics, so people with a family history of skin cancer are at higher risk. However, since non-melanoma skin cancer is so common, it frequently occurs in people who don't have a family history of the disease. Sun exposure is considered to be the main culprit.

With melanoma, genetic factors are believed to play a more major role. In 1994 a genetic mutation was discovered that researchers believe accounts for 10 percent of all melanoma cases and possibly the noninherited form of melanoma as well.

Within the category of inherited melanoma are certain genetic disorders that can greatly increase the risk. These include *dysplastic nevus syndrome* ("nevus" means "mole") and *familial atypical multiple mole melanoma syndrome* (FAM-M), which puts family members at risk for a number of malignancies, including cancers of the eye, breast, respiratory tract, gastrointestinal tract, and lymphatic system.

You are most likely to develop inherited melanoma if you have a close relative who has it, and in addition you were born with, or develop, a certain type of mole known as *atypical*. These types of moles, which may signal danger, are discussed later in this chapter.

Sun Exposure

"When I was young, my parents said, 'Get out in the sun and get some color.' Now you're told to stay indoors," says Janet, 51, putting into words precisely the dilemma that many people find themselves in today.

The rise in all forms of skin cancer has everything to do with our love affair with the sun. In the late 1800s, when women visited the seashore, they wore long skirts and gripped parasols in their hands. Alas, as we shed our inhibitions, we also shed our clothes. Today's epidemic of skin cancer can be directly traced to decades of sunbathing. It turns out that all that sun wasn't so healthy, after all.

The sun, unfortunately, is a source of radiation, which is emitted in different types of rays: UVA (ultraviolet A) and UVB (ultraviolet B) rays. Obviously, exposure to these rays causes sunburn, but there are other, less obvious effects as well.

Although the UVA rays produce less skin redness than the shorter UVB rays, these longer rays are the more damaging. These rays cause not only skin cancer but also other sun-related effects such as wrinkles and age spots. These skin changes were once thought solely due to aging, but are now recognized as the result of longtime sun exposure.

Since the shorter UVB rays are partially absorbed by the earth's ozone layer, there's concern that thinning of this atmospheric layer will cause skin cancer rates to skyrocket. But it's sunbathing, not this environmental factor, that is blamed for the current skin cancer epidemic.

A History of Past Sunburns

Sharon, a 36-year-old homemaker, was enjoying an idyllic summer in the suburbs, with two children to watch over, a flower bed filled with blooms to tend, and a brand-new outdoor pool for frequent dips. One day her daughter's teacher stopped by to chat.

"She said to me, 'Gee, I hope you're careful in the sun.' I replied, 'No, not really.' 'Well,' she continued, 'I don't mean to scare you, but I had skin cancer. You'd better be careful.'" With this, Sharon remembered a mole on her leg she'd recently noticed, and she made an appointment to see her doctor. The diagnosis was indeed skin cancer.

"I'm very fair-skinned. When I was a child in Maine, we lived on the coast. I got such bad sunburns I remember crying," Sharon recalls.

If you suffered painful or blistering sunburns in the past, you're more likely to develop skin cancer in later years. Exactly what role past sunburns play in developing melanoma isn't known, but many melanoma victims have experienced at least one severe, blistering sunburn, usually when they were children or teenagers. These episodes may have triggered changes that result in melanoma years later, often on body parts that are seldom exposed to the sun.

Light Skin and Hair Color

Your skin tone, hair color, and how your skin reacts to the sun all play a role in your susceptibility to skin cancer. The American Academy of Dermatology classifies skin into six different types, each of which has different ramifications for skin cancer. These skin types, arranged by numerical rating, are as follows. The lower the number, the higher your sensitivity to the sun.

I. Always burns easily, never tans; extremely sun-sensitive skin. Examples include people with red hair, people with freckles, Celtics, and Scots/Irish.

II. Always burns easily, tans minimally; very sun-sensitive skin. Includes fair-skinned, fair-haired, blue-eyed whites.

III. Sometimes burns, tans gradually to light brown; sun-sensitive skin. People with average skin.

IV. Burns minimally, always tan to moderate brown; minimally sun-sensitive. Mediterranean-type whites.

V. Rarely burns, tans well; sun-insensitive skin. Middle Eastern people, some Hispanics, and lighter-skinned blacks.

VI. Never burns, deeply pigmented; sun-insensitive skin. Blacks.

Beat Your Risk: *Even if you have a skin type that seldom burns, the American Academy of Dermatology recommends the daily use of sunscreen.*

Living in a Sunny Climate

For many reasons, most of us envy those who live in sunny climates—but not when it comes to skin cancer. In such places the rays of the sun are stronger, correlating with the higher rate of skin cancer. For example, Tucson, Arizona, has the highest skin cancer rate in the United States, while the number of cases in cloudy Maine is lowest, according to the National Cancer Institute. Furthermore, people who migrate to sunny places also develop a higher incidence of skin cancer. Australia, settled largely by the fair-skinned English and Irish, has the world's highest skin cancer rate.

Beat Your Risk: *It's not only the summer sun that should concern you. The sun's rays reflect powerfully—a full 80 percent—on snow. Also, even in dreary climates, ultraviolet rays can reach through the clouds. So using sunscreen year-round, no matter what the weather, is a good habit.*

HOW TO REDUCE THE RISK OF SKIN CANCER AND MELANOMA

Use Sunscreen

You've seen the ads that show women (and sometimes men) toasting on the beach. From such ads you might think that all you need to do is slather on the sunscreen and then bask in the sun with impunity. Wrong!

Even though sunscreen provides some protection against skin cancer, most people who use it stay out too long, erroneously believing that they are completely protected. So instead of being the solution, the sunscreen becomes part of the problem.

Sunscreens are protective substances that extend the length of time you can safely be outside. You can judge the protectiveness of a sunscreen according to its sun protection factor (SPF). For example, if your skin ordinarily turns pink after 10 minutes, a sunscreen with an SPF of 15 extends this to two and a half hours (10 minutes times the 15 protection factor equals 150 minutes). The American Academy of Dermatology strongly recommends using a sunscreen with an SPF reading of at least 15.

If a reading of 15 is good, isn't a higher number better? Perhaps, but it depends on your individual characteristics. For instance, if you're particularly fair-skinned, live at a high altitude where the sun's rays are stronger, or spend a lot of time outdoors, choose a sunscreen with an SPF number of 25 or 30. However, there is no evidence that a number higher than 30 provides any more protection, and it usually costs more.

Whether you apply your sunscreen in the form of a cream, oil, lotion, or gel is up to you. However, some oils have very low SPF levels. Remember, too, that although all sunscreens need to be periodically reapplied, the gels need to be reapplied more often.

Apply sunscreen generously. When it is applied too skimpily, the SPF may be one-half that advertised on the product.

A controversial study presented in 1998 at a conference of the American Association for the Advancement of Science maintained that sunscreen doesn't prevent melanoma. But other research shows it does, so the issue remains in dispute. In the meantime, the American Academy of Dermatology, concerned that people would toss out their sunscreen, issued a warning that to do so would result in an even higher skin cancer toll.

Tips for Enjoying Safe Sun

Even the strictest of experts admit that sunshine is alluring. Dr. Leftell displays a framed snapshot of his family at the beach (under a beach umbrella). Associate professor of dermatology at Yale Medical School, Dr. Jean Bolognia, also doesn't ban the sun; she advises enjoying it sparingly. "I liken sun exposure to drinking alcohol. Obviously, a glass of wine with dinner is not bad, but drinking a fifth of whiskey every night is," Dr. Bolognia said at the second annual Congress on Women's Health in 1994.

Here are some tips to reduce the odds of skin cancer:

• Limit your sun exposure between ten a.m. and three p.m., when ultraviolet rays are the strongest.

• Wear a hat with a wide brim and tightly woven clothing that covers most of your skin.

• Choose a sunscreen labeled *broad-spectrum*. This means it screens out both types of ultraviolet rays.

• Use a sunscreen year round, but especially if you're going to be outdoors for more than 20 minutes. Applying it at least 15 to 30 minutes *before* going outdoors increases its effectiveness. After swimming or doing an activity that has caused you to sweat, reapply the sunscreen. Sunscreens are not waterproof.

• Some sunscreens are alcohol-based and can sting your eyes. Choose a chemically based sunscreen instead if you're planning to play a sport such as tennis and sweat from your forehead will run into your eyes. If you're sensitive to the chemicals, try a sunblock. Sunblock agents are particularly effective because they block the widest spectrum of light, but because they are visible, they are often cosmetically unacceptable. A compound called micronized titanium dioxide provides the benefits of a physical sunblock without the white coloring.

• If you wear foundation or use a moisturizer, choose one of the many available today that have sunscreen.

• You don't have to pay for a pricey sunscreen; the inexpensive ones are as effective.

• Protect your children as well; teach them about using sunscreen.

Beat Your Risk: *We tend to think of sunscreens as something to use at the beach or when sunning ourselves. But remember that you're exposed to the sun even when you're taking a long walk. So don't forget your sunscreen then.*

Stay Out of Tanning Parlors

There's a belief that getting a tan at a tanning parlor before going on vacation provides protection. That's a myth! A sun tan is the skin's response to an injury, whether it comes from the sun or the lamps in a tanning parlor.

A 1995 study published by researchers in England in the *New England Journal of Medicine* demonstrated the harmful effects of tanning parlors. This study focused on the case of a 43-year-old woman who developed patchy, scaly skin on areas of her body not exposed to sunlight. The problem apparently was caused because the woman lay nude on an ultraviolet tanning bed once or twice a week for three years. This study was deemed important because in the past it's been difficult to single out tanning parlors as hazardous since those who use them usually sunbathe as well.

Beat Your Risk: *Back in the old days, getting a tan from a bottle meant turning your skin a fetching shade of orange. Nowadays, the sunless tanners on the store shelves will surprise you. The latest formulas are easy to use, pleasantly scented, and come in a variety of natural-looking colors to match every skin type. So this summer, enjoy a safe, sunless tan.*

Cut Down on Dietary Fat

Sun exposure is the major cause of skin cancer. But there is evidence that the harmful effect of sunlight may be accentuated by eating a high-fat diet. According to some research, animals fed a high-fat diet develop a greater number of skin cancers when they are exposed to ultraviolet light, and changing to a low-fat diet after exposure can reduce the skin cancer rate. Researchers tested this hypothesis in humans in research published in 1994 in the *New England Journal of Medicine*. Researchers divided 76 male and female skin cancer patients into two groups. One was asked to follow their customary diet, in which about 40 percent of the calories were derived from fat; the other group's intake of fat was about half that. Those who ate less fat had fewer skin cancers. Since this was a small study, more research is needed. Still, this is another reason to cut saturated fat from your diet. For information on how to do this, see chapter 16.

Screening for Skin Cancer

As of now, the best screening test for skin cancer is one you do yourself. It's called the skin self-exam. But first you need to learn about moles, which can alert you not only to skin cancer but to deadly melanoma.

"It was barely the size of a pin," recalls Rita, talking about a tiny mole she suddenly noticed on her chest. Since she worked in a medical center, she went to see a dermatologist. "It's probably nothing," the doctor said, but she ordered a biopsy anyway. This tiniest of moles did indeed turn out to be skin cancer.

Most light-skinned women have a number of small, colored, harmless-seeming spots on their bodies: moles, freckles, and birthmarks. It's estimated that the average young woman has at least twenty-five brown moles. We are usually born with a few, and the rest develop throughout our life. Most moles are normal and remain so. But in some families people have a lot of moles, and often they are abnormal. People in these families are at risk for developing melanoma.

Moles also change as we age. Adolescents and young adults tend to have dark, flat moles that become slightly elevated and begin to lose color as they age. So by the age of 80 people rarely have moles. However, mole changes that do not occur as part of the normal aging process are those that should be checked.

Beat Your Risk: Moles you've had from childhood are usually harmless. But new moles, irregularly shaped moles, and moles that undergo changes are nothing to fool around with. They must be checked by a dermatologist.

The Skin Self-Exam

Detecting potentially problematic moles should not be left to chance. Here's a method to conquer the odds that you'll find them. You're familiar with the breast self-exam. To conquer the odds of skin cancer, make the skin self-exam part of your health regimen.

To begin, stand naked before a full-length mirror. Examine your scalp, parting your hair into small segments. Look your entire body over. Check your genitals, the inside of your mouth, the backs of your ears, and the soles of your feet. Use a small hand mirror, or ask your partner, to check your back. If you find a new mole or skin marking, or if a marking apparently has grown, changed color, or looks or feels differently, contact your doctor. Remember that melanoma can appear anywhere, but in women it most commonly occurs on the arms, trunk, head, and neck, and especially the legs.

The ABC and D's of Moles

As you do your self-exam, keep in mind the National Cancer Institute's A,B,C, and D's of moles.

A—Asymmetry. An *atypical* mole is asymmetrical, which means it is irregular in shape. In other words, if you draw an imaginary line through it, you would not have matching halves. Such a mole can be a sign of trouble.

B—Border. The borders of early melanomas are usually uneven, with scalloped or notched edges.

C—Color. Moles are usually a single shade of brown, so a mole with different shades of brown or black may be the first sign of melanoma. Beware also of moles that lose color or turn white.

D—Diameter. Most harmless moles are usually less than one-quarter inch in diameter, the size of a pencil eraser. Early melanomas tend to be larger than this.

Note your moles on a diagram, and alert your doctor if you notice any new moles or suspicious changes. If you're still concerned, are at high risk for melanoma, or have lots of moles, consider going to a dermatologist and having your moles "mapped." If a mole does appear suspicious, it will be biopsied and sent to a lab for analysis.

Beat Your Risk: *To get into the habit of doing a skin self-exam, do it on the same day of your monthly breast self-exam.*

THE BOTTOM LINE

Investigate your family history to determine if skin cancer or melanoma runs in your family. If you believe you have a rare genetic skin cancer or melanoma syndrome, contact your dermatologist. Be aware of the moles you have and do a monthly self-exam, keeping the A,B,C, and D's of moles in mind.

Rate Your Risk: Skin Cancer

Put a check mark after each answer. Answer all questions. Then consult the scoring key to compute your score.

Score

	(+ column)	(– column)
Family History		
1. Have you a parent, brother, sister or child who has been treated for skin cancer or melanoma?		
Yes____ +1 No ____ 0		
2. What is your race?		
White +5		
African-American +1		
Other light-skinned racial group +3		
Other dark-skinned racial group +2		
3. Do you have fair skin, freckles, or red hair?		
Yes____ +3 No ____ 0		
4. Do you live in a part of the country that is sunny most of the year?		
Yes____ +5 No ____ 0		
5. During warm weather, do you often stay out in the sun long enough to burn or tan?		
Yes____ +3 No ____ 0		

6. In your work, are you outside most of the day?

   Yes_____ +2   No _____ 0

7. Do you take part in outdoor sports or other activities where you can get a sunburn or suntan?

   Yes_____ +2   No _____ 0

8. Do you sunbathe to get a tan?

   Yes_____ +3   No _____ 0

9. If you wore no sunscreen and you stayed out in strong sunlight for the first time in summer, you would:

   Get a severe, blistering sunburn   +3

   Get a mild burn followed by some tanning   +2

   Get brown without any sunburn   +1

10. Do you always use sunscreen of 15 SPF or greater in the summer?

    Yes_____ −1   No _____ +2

11. Do you use a sunscreen of 15 SPF or greater in the winter?

    Yes_____ −1   No _____ +1

12. How many moles do you have?

    Very few   0

    5 to 30   +1

    31 to 100   +2

    More than 100   +3

13. Do you have any moles that are irregular in shape or color?

    Yes_____ +3   No _____ 0

14. Have you ever had a malignant mole removed from your skin?

    Yes_____ +3   No _____ 0

15. Do you now, or did you in the past,   _____ _____
    use a sun-tanning parlor?
    Yes_____ +3   No _____ 0
    Subtotal   _____
    Risk Factor   +5
    (add in only if you answered
    yes to all or either #1, 8, 13, 14, or 15)
    Final Score   _____

How to Score

1. Fill in the numbers in the columns at the far right.
2. Subtotal your score from the plus and minus columns.
3. Add the +5 if you answered yes to particular risk factors.
4. Compute your final score.
5. Compare your score to the Risk Factor Scoring Chart.

Skin Cancer Risk Factor Scoring Chart

Below 8   Lowest risk
9 to 16   Low to moderate
17 to 24   Moderate to high
Above 25   Highest risk

11

DIABETES

I F YOU READ THE OBITUARIES, you'll find such causes of death as "heart disease," "kidney disease," or "stroke." Rarely is diabetes mentioned. You may remain unaware, unless you've experienced the damage diabetes does to your body, or experienced it through a loved one, that diabetes can set the stage for these major ailments.

Ethel was 62 when she had her heart attack one morning after she arrived at her job where she worked as a credit manager. "I felt hot and I couldn't talk. I had pain in my chest," she recalls. In the hospital she learned she was diabetic. "I hadn't seen a doctor in twenty years," she said. Since then she's learned that "having 'sugar' is quite common," she said, using a common name for diabetes. "But I didn't know I had sugar," she added. "I had no symptoms." Diabetes also occurs in women younger than Ethel; one of her daughters has the disease as well.

An estimated 16 million Americans, over half of them women, have diabetes. About 150,000 die annually from complications of this disease, making it the nation's fourth leading killer. As we age, the number of diabetes cases will increase.

What is frightening is that half of those who have diabetes don't realize it. On average there is a seven-year gap between the onset and the diagnosis of the disease. During this time diabetes silently damages the blood vessels of the body, from the eyes to the toes, and all of the organs in between.

WHAT IS DIABETES?

Diabetes is a metabolic disorder in which the body's ability to manufacture insulin is diminished. Insulin is a crucial hormone that enables blood sugar to enter the body's cells to be used for energy. Diabetes also results in an elevated level of glucose, or sugar, in the blood, which damages the cells. Since the cells are the basic unit of life, diabetes ultimately affects the entire body.

Diabetics are at greatly increased risk for the following ailments:

High blood pressure. People with diabetes are twice as likely to develop high blood pressure.

Heart disease. Diabetes leads to atherosclerosis, the dangerous narrowing of the heart's coronary arteries, which causes heart attacks. Although deadly to men's hearts, diabetes is even more damaging to women's. Diabetic women also develop heart disease earlier than nondiabetic women.

Stroke. Diabetes injuries the delicate blood vessels in the brain, increasing the probability of a stroke.

Kidney disease. Diabetes causes the kidneys to work too hard, causing kidney disease in 10 percent of diabetics. Ultimately the kidneys may be destroyed, leading to the need for dialysis, a kidney transplant, or death.

Blindness. Because diabetes damages the tiny capillaries in the eyes, diabetics are 25 times more likely than nondiabetics to lose their sight. This complication occurs more often in female diabetics.

Nerve damage. Approximately 50 percent of all diabetics develop nerve damage, which can lead to loss of feeling, muscular weakness, and, quite often, the amputation of a leg or foot. Female diabetics are especially more likely to develop *peripheral vascular disease* (PVD), which causes pain in the thighs, calves, and buttocks, and is associated with increased risk of coronary heart disease, stroke, and heart failure.

Pancreatic cancer. Although not usually considered a complication of diabetes, people with diabetes are at increased risk of developing this deadly, quick-killing type of cancer, some studies find.

How can you avoid these complications? The best way is to reduce your risk of developing diabetes in the first place.

Conquer the Odds: *Sometimes people are told that they have a "mild" form of diabetes. Even mildly elevated glucose levels caused by diabetes can damage your body, so if you've been told you have mild diabetes, learn to strictly control it.*

THE TYPES OF DIABETES

There are generally considered to be two types of diabetes. The first, Type I, affects only a relatively small number of people. Type II accounts for a whopping 90 percent of all cases. A third type, gestational diabetes, which occurs during pregnancy and can endanger the health of the unborn child, is discussed later on.

Type I Diabetes

This was once known as *juvenile onset* diabetes because most (but not all) cases develop in childhood. This type of the disease is characterized by destruction of the cells in the pancreas that produce insulin. It has two forms. *Immune-mediated diabetes mellitus* results from an autoimmune response in the body, possibly to a virus. It typically strikes children or slim adults, but it can arise at any age. *Idiopathic Type I diabetes* is a rare form of the disease that has no known cause.

Type II Diabetes

Diabetics with this form of the disease do produce insulin, but the amount may be diminished, and their bodies are unable to use it properly. It typically occurs in people over the age of 45 who have other risk factors for the disease, as discussed later.

It's believed there is a genetic link between these two major types of diabetes, because children who develop Type I diabetes often come from a family with a history of Type II diabetes. But not all the answers about either type are known, and more research needs to be done.

This book is primarily concerned with showing you how to prevent Type II diabetes, because it is by far the most common form and, unlike Type I, is preventable. So Type II diabetes is simply referred to as diabetes for the remainder of this chapter.

FACTORS THAT INCREASE YOUR RISK OF DIABETES

Growing Older

Diabetes develops most often after the age of 40, although it can develop earlier.

Race

Women of all races develop diabetes, but African-American women develop it far more often and also when they are younger. Latina women are also at higher than average risk. Some groups of Native Americans, particularly the Pima Indians of Arizona, have an extremely high rate of diabetes, although they also tend to escape some of the complications, such as heart disease, a fact that puzzles researchers. Some studies also have found Asians to be at higher than average risk.

Family Medical History

Although genetics plays a role in who develops diabetes, it is much less predictable than such strictly inherited diseases as Huntington's disease, which is handed down directly from parent to child. So although having a family history increases your risk of diabetes, it is impossible to predict which family members it will strike. But the more relatives who have it, the greater your risk is.

Furthermore, people within families tend to develop diabetes at widely varying ages. With most forms of cancer, developing it at a younger than average age is often an indication of heredity at work. Not so with diabetes; heredity may be at work in a woman who gets diabetes at 40, even if her only other affected relative was her grand-mother, who wasn't diagnosed as a diabetic until she was 70.

Obesity

If you are overweight, the likelihood that you will become dia-betic soars. This is especially true if you have diabetes in your family history; however, gaining weight in middle age increases your risk of diabetes even if you have no relatives with the disease. This is true even for those who gain only a small amount of weight, although the more weight gained, the higher the risk. The good news is, if you lose weight as you grow older, your risk of becoming diabetic de-creases, according to findings based on 114,281 women enrolled in the Nurses' Health Study that were published in 1995 in the *Annals of Internal Medicine*.

These findings call into question the belief that gaining a small amount of weight as women age is advisable and to be expected. "From the public health standpoint, the message should be to women that they should avoid gaining the excess weight that can come from child-bearing and going through menopause," says Dr. JoAnn Manson, co-investigator of the Nurses' Health Study.

Does it matter where this extra weight is situated? The risk of de-veloping diabetes is greater for apple-shaped women who carry their excess weight in their midriff, most experts believe. Although the exact reason for this is not known, it is believed that abdominal fat interferes with the body's ability to use insulin efficiently. Still, if you are fat enough, you may get diabetes, no matter how your weight is distributed.

Another potential marker for diabetes is having little skin "tags" on your body—little nubs of redundant skin that are sometimes seen on heavy women. These little malformations are tangible signs of insulin resistance and may be a warning sign prior to symptoms developing.

Sedentary Lifestyle

No matter whether you are thin or heavy, being inactive increases the risk of diabetes. Several studies show that even if your family history predisposes you to diabetes, if you stay physically active, you'll reduce that risk. Also, although the Nurses' Health Study found obesity increased the diabetes risk for middle-aged women, some experts who viewed the study say the culprit may instead be inactivity.

It used to be believed that women who gave birth to several children were likely to develop diabetes. Women who gave birth to several children are more likely to develop diabetes, but this may be due to the fact that they are also more likely to be overweight.

High Blood Pressure

Although it isn't known precisely why, having high blood pressure increases the probability of developing diabetes.

Smoking

Although smoking is not considered a major risk factor for diabetes, it may be a contributor and/or increase the risk of complications. A Harvard School of Public Health study published in 1995 in the *British Medical Journal* found that middle-aged men who smoked more than 25 cigarettes a day doubled their diabetes risk. Two years earlier, the Nurses' Health Study had found similar results. According to this study, published in the *American Journal of Public Health*, current female smokers had a higher diabetes risk, and the heavier the smoking, the higher the risk. Exactly how smoking raises the risk of diabetes isn't known, but smokers tend to have higher blood glucose levels and increased insulin resistance, both contributing factors to the disease.

A History of Gestational Diabetes

When Janet was pregnant with her first baby, she gained "a whopping 55 pounds," she recalls. Previously slender, she had always grappled with a weight problem. Her first son was born large but healthy. Janet neglected to lose all her "baby fat," but the second time around, she watched her weight more carefully. Despite this she developed gestational diabetes. "I had to follow a strict diet and monitor my blood glucose levels three times a day. It was no picnic," she recalls. Janet's diligence paid off, and she delivered a healthy baby girl. Now she says, "I'm making sure I lose all that extra weight."

Gestational diabetes occurs only in pregnant women. This form of diabetes, which occurs in an estimated 2 to 4 percent of all pregnant women, disappears soon after birth.

Gestational diabetes increases the risk of:

- The infant dying within the first month after birth
- Developing pregnancy-related hypertension, a dangerous condition also known as toxemia
- Delivering a large birth-weight baby, which can injure mothers of small builds

Happily, these problems can be avoided if gestational diabetes is diagnosed and properly controlled. If you're at higher than average risk for diabetes, you should be tested for gestational diabetes as soon as you become pregnant.

There are wide variations in the prevalence of gestational diabetes among racial and ethnic groups. It more commonly occurs in African-American women and Latinas, although white women develop it too. Controlling gestational diabetes is important for all women but is particularly crucial for African-American women, whose babies are extremely sensitive to the effects of too much glucose during gestation, according to Lois Jovanovic, M.D., a California endocrinologist who specializes in the treatment of gestational diabetes.

Overweight women are at higher risk, but slender women can develop gestational diabetes as well.

If You Had Gestational Diabetes, Will You Get Diabetes Later?

"My grandmother had diabetes and I had gestational diabetes, so there's nothing I can do about it," declared Marianne, a TV producer. Her fatalistic attitude is all too common, but it's wrong. Although the majority of these women—about 60 percent—do become diabetic later in life, there are ways to avoid it, according to Dr. Jovanovic. She noted that a study demonstrated that one such group of women were able to cut their risk by losing weight. Those who were most successful were able to change from at high to low risk, she said.

According to Dr. Jovanovic, women with gestational diabetes who may develop diabetes later in life are those who:

• Were obese at the time their gestational diabetes was diagnosed
• Have a high fasting reading on their glucose tolerance test at the time of their pregnancy
• Must take insulin during pregnancy to control their diabetes
• Have glucose levels that do not return to normal after birth

---

Beat Your Risk: If you've had gestational diabetes, be sure to have your glucose tested after your baby is born. If you fall into one of the groups with a higher than average risk of developing diabetes later on, see an endocrinologist who specializes in diabetes so you can take action to lower your risk.

Impaired Glucose Homeostasis: The "Red Flag" of Diabetes

Research is increasingly focusing on the years when a woman begins developing diabetes and when her blood glucose level rises high enough to be classified as diabetic. This midway condition, known as *impaired glucose homeostasis*, signifies that the body is no longer secreting and/or using insulin properly. Two categories of impaired glucose homeostasis are considered risk factors for future diabetes: *impaired fasting glucose* (IFG) and the more severe *impaired glucose tol-*

erance (IGT). These categories reflect the amount of fasting plasma in the blood and are diagnosed by the use of glucose tolerance tests, which are explained later in this chapter.

Prior to 1997, IGT was the only category. The American Diabetes Association added the category after research demonstrated that people with this condition were also at high risk of developing diabetes and blood vessel complications, such as heart attacks and strokes. The Association recommends that people falling into these categories be tested more often for the onset of diabetes. A large-scale study to determine if early treatment can prevent or delay the development of diabetes in people with these conditions is now underway.

So if you are diagnosed with impaired glucose homeostasis, it should be an important motivation to conquer the odds. "It is a red flag. It means you need to get going and change your lifestyle," says Kathleen Wishner, M.D., president of the American Diabetes Association.

OTHER POSSIBLE RISK FACTORS

Oral Contraceptives

When oral contraceptives were first developed, they were found to affect glucose metabolism adversely, so diabetics and women who had developed gestational diabetes were warned not to take them. But a new pill that has been developed, composed of a synthetic progestin called *norgestimate*, can be taken by these women. So if you fall into these categories, and you want to take the Pill, ask your doctor about it.

What about Hypoglycemia?

Since the definition of diabetes is having a high blood sugar level, it was thought that those who were hypoglycemic, meaning they had too low a level of sugar in their blood, would inevitably develop diabetes eventually. However, this is no longer the case.

First, the number of people who are truly hypoglycemic is smaller than you may think. "Hypoglycemia was a fad diagnosis ten years ago," says Dr. Jovanovic. It's now believed that what appeared to be low blood sugar is actually a normal variation in how some people metabolize their food.

The problem arises from the fact that the test for hypoglycemia involves fasting and then downing a sugary drink. Under these circumstances, 40 percent of people tested four hours after taking the sugar drink will be classified as hypoglycemic, even those who are perfectly healthy. Symptoms of panic disorder or anxiety, like a racing pulse and becoming jittery, can also be mistaken for hypoglycemia. There may be a small percentage of true hypoglycemics, but the number is far smaller than previously believed.

However, some women who are in the process of becoming diabetic may produce too much insulin and may experience symptoms, such as shakiness, that can be mistaken for hypoglycemia.

HOW TO REDUCE THE RISK OF DIABETES

In the past, preventing diabetes hasn't been emphasized, but this attitude is changing as the rate of diabetes climbs and evidence grows that it is one of the most preventable ailments. Indeed, some experts estimate that up to a whopping 80 percent of diabetes could be prevented by changes in lifestyle, primarily losing weight and exercising. Furthermore, if you successfully stave off developing diabetes, you've dramatically lowered your risk of heart disease and stroke, two major killers of women.

You can greatly reduce your risk of becoming diabetic by slimming down. Alas, that's often easier said than done. Most women who become diabetic also have a tendency to gain weight and find it difficult to lose. However, even a modest weight loss, such as 20 or 30 pounds, can improve the blood sugar levels in someone who is, say, 50 to 100 pounds overweight or even more, experts say. So even if you have a lot of weight to lose, don't be discouraged. Follow the healthy eating principles outlined later in this book. Bear in mind that exercise is also extremely important if you seek to reduce your risk of becoming diabetic.

Exercise

It's well established that exercise can help diabetics control their disease. What's becoming overwhelmingly apparent is that exercise can also help keep women from developing it in the first place.

The Nurses' Health Study found that women who participated in regular, vigorous exercise cut their risk of developing diabetes by a third. This included even those women with a family history of the disease. "This is a finding that has been confirmed by additional studies, and the link between exercise and the prevention of diabetes makes biological sense," says Dr. Manson. Diabetics, and those prone to develop it, are "insulin resistant." Exercise counteracts this problem because when you're active, your body uses insulin more efficiently.

In fact, exercise has been shown to help the body compensate for faulty insulin metabolism. When you exercise, your body creates new insulin receptors. But this effect is only temporary. To maintain it, you need to exercise on a consistent basis and have it really become part of your lifestyle.

What type of exercise is best for preventing diabetes? Cardiovascular exercise is recommended. Also important for those who are prone to diabetes is muscle-building, says Dr. Richard Bernstein, who has authored several books on diabetes. He's found that people who do strength-training exercises, replacing fat with muscle, metabolize insulin more efficiently.

Beat Your Risk: In the past there has not been enough emphasis on preventing diabetes, and some doctors still may not place much importance on it. So if you are at risk for diabetes, and your doctor brushes off your concern, be persistent.

Screening for Diabetes

Because diabetes can greatly damage the body before it is detected, the American Diabetes Association has called for broader screening. Under guidelines adopted in 1997, all adults, not only those at risk for the disease, should be screened for diabetes beginning at the age of 45. If the results are normal, the screening test should be repeated every three years thereafter.

Adults with risk factors, the Association recommends, should first be screened at a younger age and retested more often. These risk factors are:

- Being overweight (more than 20 percent above ideal body weight)
- Having a first-degree relative (parent or sibling) with diabetes
- Being a member of a high-risk ethnic population (African-American, Latina, Native American, Asian)
- Delivering a baby weighing more than nine pounds or having been diagnosed with gestational diabetes
- Having high blood pressure
- Having unfavorable blood cholesterol levels
- Being found to have IFG or IGT in previous testing

There are three different ways to screen for diabetes:

Fasting Plasma Glucose Test

In 1997 the American Diabetes Association declared this the preferred screening test. It is a simple blood test that measures the amount of glucose in the blood following an eight-hour fast. It used to be that a level of 140 milligrams per deciliter on this test signified diabetes; however, that level has been lowered to 126 in hopes of identifying diabetics earlier, before complications set in.

Casual Plasma Glucose Test

This is a simple blood test that can be done anytime, regardless of meals.

Oral Glucose Tolerance Test

Prior to 1997, this was the recommended test; however, the ADA has since decided it is too cumbersome for regular screening. It is now used as a diagnostic test when symptoms of diabetes exist. For this test you drink a liquid with glucose in it, and blood is taken every thirty minutes for two hours while you rest. A reading of more than 200 milligrams per deciliter between zero and two hours and at two hours indicates diabetes.

The results of these tests can be influenced by factors such as the taking of certain drugs, the significant restriction of carbohydrate intake, low potassium levels, stress, and prolonged inactivity, so the test should be redone to confirm the results.

Generally two abnormal results using any of these three tests—on two different days—are required to make a diagnosis of diabetes.

Beat Your Risk: *If you are developing diabetes, finding out as early as possible is critically important. So if your blood glucose level begins creeping up over 110 milligrams per deciliter, make sure your doctor puts you on a screening program.*

Screening for Gestational Diabetes

If you're pregnant, or plan to be, you need to know about screening for gestational diabetes. Previously, all pregnant women were screened for the disease. The 1997 guidelines now recommend that all pregnant women be screened in their third trimester with the exception of women who meet *all* of the following criteria:

- Less than 25 years old
- Normal body weight
- No family history of diabetes
- Not a member of an ethnic group with a higher prevalence of diabetes (Latina, Native American, African-American, Asian)

Beat Your Risk: *In the past, a simple urine sample, known as a urinalysis, was sometimes used to screen for diabetes. This is not a useful screening tool because once the glucose level is high enough to spill into the urine, the disease probably has been present for years.*

Know the Diabetes Warning Signs

What follows are warning signs that you may have diabetes. Remember that spotting warning signs as general as thirst can be tricky. Says Josie, a West Indian woman in her late sixties, "It was a hot summer, so I didn't realize I was spending all my time by the sink, drinking glasses of water."

Furthermore, unexplained weight loss can be cause for concern. A writer in her thirties developed Type I diabetes after her second baby was born. She was unaware of it, though. In fact, she was lavishly praised by her relatives, her friends, and even the doctor's nurse because she was steadily losing weight. She was delighted because she wasn't even dieting. Not until she nearly collapsed into a diabetic coma did she realize something was very wrong.

Beat Your Risk: *Remember that even though Type I diabetes was once known as juvenile onset diabetes, it can strike at any age.*

Warning signs of Type I diabetes are:

- Frequent urination
- Unusual thirst
- Extreme hunger
- Unexplained weight loss
- Extreme fatigue
- Irritability

Warning signs of Type II diabetes are:

- Any of the warning symptoms listed for Type I diabetes
- Frequent or recurring infections, such as skin, gum, or urinary tract
- Blurred vision
- Cuts and bruises that heal slowly
- Tingling or numbness in the hands or feet

Remember, while the symptoms of Type I diabetes tend to come on suddenly, the warning signs of Type II diabetes can be more subtle. Ethel, a 62-year-old woman, didn't realize that she had diabetes until she suffered a heart attack. "I hadn't been to a doctor in twenty years. I was never sick, and I don't like doctors," she says. After her heart attack, she learned she had both diabetes and high blood pressure. This is not surprising. Diabetes can be silent. Conventionally, you think of women with diabetes as having warning signs, such as extreme thirst, frequent urination, and weight loss. But you may have no symptoms at all. This is why diabetes is so insidious.

THE FUTURE

The National Institutes of Health have launched a major clinical trial to find ways of preventing diabetes. The study will involve about 3,000 participants at 23 sites across the country. One group will be treated with weight control and exercise; the other will be given a drug believed to reduce insulin levels. The result will hopefully result in more emphasis on effective ways to prevent diabetes in the future.

THE BOTTOM LINE

Although its significance is seldom recognized, diabetes is one of the greatest—and most preventable—health problems for women. If you are at risk for diabetes, because of either family medical history or being overweight, take a proactive stance and talk to your doctor about undergoing the screening tests outlined in this chapter. No matter what the results, change your lifestyle. Eat healthy, and get moving!

Rate Your Risk: Diabetes

Put a check mark after each answer. Answer all questions. Then consult the scoring key to compute your score.

		Score	
		(+ column)	(– column)

Family History

1. Do you have any close relatives who have diabetes?
   Yes_____ +1   No _____ 0

2. Do you have more than two close relatives in your family who have diabetes?
   Yes_____ +2   No _____ 0

3. What race are you?
   White   +1
   Hispanic   +2
   African-American   +2
   Other   +1

Personal History/Habits

4. What is your age?
   39 or less _____ 0
   40 or more _____ +1

5. Do you weigh more than 20 pounds over your ideal weight?
   Yes_____ +2   No _____ 0

6. Do you have high blood pressure
   Yes_____ +2   No _____ 0

7. Do you smoke?
   Yes_____ +1   No _____ 0

8. If you were ever pregnant, did you develop gestational diabetes?
   Yes_____ +1   No _____ 0

9. Are you generally inactive?   _____ _____

   Yes_____ +1   No _____ 0

10. Do you exercise at least 30 minutes a   _____ _____

    day three days a week or more?

    Yes_____ −1   No _____ 0

        Subtotal   _____

        Risk Factor   +5

        (add in only if you answered

        yes to all or either #2 or 5)

        Final Score   _____

How to Score

1. Fill in the numbers in the columns at the far right.

2. Subtotal your score from the plus and minus columns.

3. Add the +5 if you answered yes to particular risk factors.

4. Compute your final score.

5. Compare your score to the Risk Factor Scoring Chart.

Diabetes Risk Factor Scoring Chart

   4 or below   Lowest risk

   5 to 9   Low to moderate

   10 to 14   Moderate to high

   Above 15   Highest risk

CHAPTER 12

HEART DISEASE

A SUCCESSFUL BUSINESSWOMAN, Rebecca was 37 when she suffered a heart attack. She'd complained about chest pain for over a year, but doctors told her that her problem was stress, brought on, undoubtedly, by her work. She was told this by doctor after doctor. Some suggested her chest pain was in her imagination; one recommended she see a psychiatrist. As the pain worsened and grew more frequent, Rebecca alternated between anger and despair. Finally, one evening, months later, while she was dining out with her friends, the pain became unbearable.

"My friends were frightened and drove me to the nearest hospital. I told the nurse I was having a heart attack. I can still see the look of disbelief on her face," Rebecca angrily recalls.

She was left alone on an examining table. Rebecca's heartbeat stopped, she went into cardiac arrest, and she fell to the floor. Fortunately, she was discovered in time and revived. But she remains understandably bitter. "No one believed me—no one, and I nearly died."

Rebecca's story is not unusual. Although heart disease is the biggest killer of women, countless women continue to be misdiagnosed and ignored. It's not known how many die or suffer crippling damage to their hearts.

Here are the facts:

- Cardiovascular disease, which is heart disease and stroke combined, kills about 470,000 American women every year. That's almost twice the number of women who die from all forms of cancer combined.
- Heart disease kills about 240,000 women annually. That's five times the number of women who die of breast cancer.
- Almost twice as many women as men die within a year after having a heart attack.

"Heart disease is far and away the major cause of all death in women. It really swamps other causes," says Dr. JoAnn Manson.

Yet heart disease in women is grievously overlooked. As a result, four out of every five women don't know that heart disease is their leading cause of death. Even more worrisome, neither do one-third of their doctors, a Gallup survey found.

The result can be tragic. Too often, women are sent home from the doctor's office, told they're suffering from "nerves" or indigestion, and are properly diagnosed only when they suffer a heart attack. Even when they are diagnosed correctly, some studies find they are less likely to be offered the same life-saving cardiac procedures, such as angioplasty or cardiac bypass surgery, as men.

Because women's hearts were erroneously assumed to be less vulnerable, research was done primarily on men, and cardiac procedures were created for them. Risk factors in men are emphasized while those more common in women, including diabetes and abdominal obesity, are ignored.

Nowadays, doctors supposedly know better. But now, even though it's more widely recognized that women do die of heart disease, it is too often mistakenly assumed that these women are in their seventies or eighties. Not necessarily.

Consider Rhoda, for example. I first met Rhoda when she interviewed me on the subject of women and heart disease for her Connecticut weekend radio show. She was trim and energetic, and although she was in her early sixties, she looked at least a decade younger. Afterward, she confided in me that she wanted to talk with me again because she'd just been diagnosed with heart disease.

"I'm very aware of breast cancer, but I had no idea that I could get heart disease," Rhoda said. Less than a week later, I received a call from her station manager, who was in tears. That Wednesday night, while dining out at a Manhattan restaurant with her husband, Rhoda had suffered a massive heart attack and died.

WHAT IS HEART DISEASE?

Heart disease is actually an umbrella term that encompasses many different maladies, including congestive heart failure, congenital heart defects, and malfunctioning heart valves. This chapter refers specifically to the kind known as coronary heart disease, also called *atherosclerosis*—the disease process that narrows the heart's coronary arteries and results in heart attack. For the purposes of simplification, this type of problem will be termed heart disease throughout this book.

WHAT CAUSES HEART DISEASE?

Heart disease is a progressive process. The first stage is often an injury to the inner lining of one of the arteries. What causes this initial injury is not known; one possible culprit is the inflammation caused by an infection, possibly a virus. But it is also believed to result from the damaging effects of risk factors such as toxins from cigarette smoke, high blood pressure, diabetes, or dangerous cholesterol. Whatever the reason, as the tissue tries to heal itself, it forms a combination of overgrown tissue, immune cells, and fat, known as plaque. This disease process is known as atherosclerosis. As the plaque accumulates beneath the artery's lining, the artery becomes narrower and narrower. If the blood supply is squeezed off, or a blood clot forms and blocks it, the result is a heart attack.

THE IMPORTANCE OF RISK FACTORS

For heart disease, identifying your risk factors is critically important. At least half of all cases of heart disease are attributable to known risk factors. This is a large number when you consider that the same can be said for only a small fraction of breast cancer cases.

Furthermore, with heart disease, the more risk factors you have, the greater your probability of a heart attack. Indeed, although in the past women were erroneously thought to be at less risk of heart disease than men, in some cases they may be in even more jeopardy.

"A fifty-five-year-old woman who smokes and has elevated cholesterol and high blood pressure has roughly three times the normal risk for a heart attack, whereas a man of the same age with the same risk factors has only twice the normal risk," says Fredric J. Pashkow, M.D., associate director of preventative cardiology and rehabilitation at the Cleveland Clinic Foundation.

Risk factors for heart disease are generally divided into two categories: *nonmodifiable* and *modifiable*. Nonmodifiable risk factors are those that cannot be changed—mainly, growing older, race, and family medical history. All the rest of the risk factors are considered modifiable. These include being overweight, smoking, and being inactive, as well as risk factors that can be controlled, including high blood pressure and diabetes. The reason for this categorization is to emphasize that even if you have nonmodifiable risk factors for heart disease, there are a great many more that you can change.

Lifestyle changes, including quitting smoking, losing weight, exercising, and taking replacement hormones, can sharply cut the rate of heart disease in women. "Studies have shown that women who quit smoking cut their heart disease rate by 65 percent. They cut their risk by 45 percent by maintaining a healthy weight, and, by being active, by 35 to 40 percent. So even though they seem simple, lifestyle changes are themselves tremendously important," says Dr. Manson.

FACTORS THAT INCREASE YOUR RISK OF HEART DISEASE

Growing Older

As you age, your risk of heart disease rises. Women generally are blessed with what is termed *gender protection*, which means they customarily develop heart disease at least 10 to 15 years later than men. Therefore, the risk for women begins to mount when they reach 50 to 55 instead of 40 to 45 for men. But after menopause, the risk begins to rise. By the time a woman reaches 75, her risk of dying from heart disease is equal to that of a man's.

This gender protection was erroneously assumed to provide women with immunity to heart disease, and in the not so distant past, this assumption was even taught in medical schools. Alternatively, student doctors were taught that if a woman did develop heart disease, it was a rare event, and she was most likely very old. This is not true! Although it is less common, women in their fifties, forties, and even thirties can develop heart disease.

Race

Heart disease is the biggest killer of women, no matter what their race or ethnic group. However, for most of their lives African-American women are more vulnerable; they are about one-third more likely to die of the disease. Between the ages of 35 and 74, they have double the risk. This difference evens out by age 75, when an equal number of white women are afflicted.

This is believed to be because African-American women are more likely to develop multiple risk factors for heart disease, including high blood pressure, diabetes, and obesity, at a younger age. Furthermore, many African-American women are poor, which bars them from receiving good medical care.

Family Medical History

"My mother died of heart disease, and I suffered my heart attack the very day after I buried her," recalls Dora, who is a receptionist at a cardiac rehabilitation center. Her aunt was only 42 when she died of a heart attack, and her grandmother succumbed to heart disease as well.

Genetics indeed, play a role in heart disease. According to a Swedish study of twins reported in 1994 in the *New England Journal of Medicine*, the link between genetics and heart disease in men is strong, but in women it's apparently stronger. The men whose identical twin died of heart disease before the age of 55 had an eightfold risk of this ailment; for fraternal twins, the risk was weaker but still nearly fourfold. Women whose fraternal twins had died had two to three times the risk of the men but for identical twins the risk was fifteen times higher.

Some of this increased risk might be due to inheriting a contributing underlying disease, such as diabetes or abnormal blood cholesterol patterns. Lifestyle may also play a role, since twins are raised in the same environment.

If you have a family history of heart disease, the age at which your relatives developed it offers a very important clue to your own risk. If your relatives developed heart disease at a relatively young age, this increases your risk. This is the case if your father or brother(s) was diagnosed before the age of 55; and/or your mother or sister(s) was diagnosed before the age of 65. What about grandparents, aunts, and cousins? Their history of the disease increases your risk, but far less so than first-degree relatives.

Remember, though, that heredity is not necessarily destiny. These findings indicate a tendency, not a certainty. Use your knowledge of a negative family medical history to motivate you to make the necessary changes that can tip the odds back in your favor.

High Blood Pressure

High blood pressure, clinically known as *hypertension*, increases your heart disease risk. This is a particularly insidious problem because it has no symptoms and damages your heart without your being aware of it.

Your heart acts as a pump that operates under a pressure system. Pressures that are too high damage the coronary arteries, the important vessels that bring blood to the heart. This damage can result in a heart attack.

Controlling high blood pressure can reduce its threat to your heart. Sometimes weight loss, exercise, and dietary changes are enough to control it, but often medication is needed.

Because high blood pressure often occurs without symptoms, having your blood pressure checked regularly is critically important. Since this is always a part of a doctor's physical examination, it's a good reason to get regular checkups.

Beat Your Risk: When your blood pressure is taken, a manually pumped blood-pressure cuff is used. There are two sizes of cuffs: one that is average-sized, and a larger one. If a cuff that is too small is used, you may be diagnosed erroneously with high blood pressure. One-time readings in pharmacies or at health fairs may also give an inaccurate picture. Bear in mind that some people become anxious in a medical office, causing a rise in blood pressure, known as white-coat *hypertension. So if your blood-pressure reading is elevated, make sure these possible causes are ruled out.*

Diabetes

Diabetes damages the heart's coronary arteries, causing heart disease. When diabetes occurs prior to menopause, it erases the "gender protection" that premenopausal women ordinarily have against heart disease.

Female diabetics with heart disease fare worse not only after heart attacks but also after procedures to treat heart disease, including coronary bypass surgery and angioplasty. Furthermore, diabetes causes nerve damage, which can mask chest pain, an important warning sign of a heart attack.

Certain risk factors have a more adverse impact when they occur together because they seem to act synergistically. The three that seem to go together, particularly in women, to raise the risk of heart disease dramatically are diabetes, high blood pressure, and a high triglyceride level. The combination of these three factors is some-times known as *syndrome* X. Having these three diseases heightens the risk of heart disease.

Beat Your Risk: *If you have diabetes, ask your doctor to monitor you to make certain you do not develop heart disease or to assess its progression if you do. This is a serious concern; make certain it's taken seriously.*

Smoking

Most people are aware that smoking causes lung cancer, but they often don't realize the strong link between cigarettes and heart dis-ease as well. But ample evidence attests to this.

First, although, as noted, most women develop heart disease 10 to 15 years later than men, smoking erases this natural gender protection. Smoking is devastating to your heart no matter what your age.

Smoking has also been found to contribute to the development of early heart disease. A study of 105 apparently healthy women in their thirties and forties found that those with signs of early heart disease were much more likely to be smokers, it was reported at a 1995 American Heart Association meeting.

Studies also find that female smokers have nearly double the heart attack rate and are more likely to suffer from advanced heart disease than nonsmokers.

Furthermore, heavy smokers are not the only ones at risk; light smokers are as well. It's been found that smoking just four cigarettes a day increases heart disease risk.

It's believed that smoking damages the heart in three major ways:

- First, the poisons in cigarette smoke apparently damage the coronary arteries.
- Second, female smokers are more likely to experience car-diac spasms—dangerous constrictions of the heart's blood vessels that can result in a heart attack—even in the absence of heart disease.

- Third, tobacco smoke increases the activity of clotting agents, which can contribute to a heart attack.

Beat Your Risk: *Don't switch to filtered or low-tar cigarettes to save your heart; these are also hazardous, possibly even more so because women may smoke more of them in the erroneous belief they are safer. And don't switch to cigars—these are also very dangerous for the heart.*

Oral Contraceptives (If You Smoke)

Oral contraceptives are considered generally safe for most women—but not for smokers. This is because the nicotine in cigarettes and oral contraceptives independently increase clotting activity, raising the risk of a heart attack up to 39 times, the American Heart Association estimates. Low-estrogen pills may lower this risk, but to what extent is not yet known

---

Beat Your Risk: *If you smoke and already have heart disease, quit. Smoking increases your risk of a heart attack. Furthermore, if you should need to undergo coronary bypass surgery, being a smoker will slow your recovery and increase the likelihood that the bypass will eventually fail.*

Abnormal Cholesterol Patterns

What Is Cholesterol?

There are two forms of cholesterol. Cholesterol can be found in some of the foods you eat, and it is also a component of your blood. Cholesterol is a vital component the body needs to form cell membranes, some hormones, and other needed tissue. But these fat substances in the blood, known as *lipids*, also contribute to the formation of the deposits known as plaque, which, as noted earlier, causes atherosclerosis, or heart disease.

Cholesterol and other lipids can't dissolve in the blood. They have to be transported to and from the cells by special carriers of lipids and proteins called *lipoproteins*. There are several types, but the ones that traditionally have garnered the most concern are low-density lipoprotein (LDL), high-density lipoprotein (HDL), and triglycerides.

Low-density lipoprotein, or LDL cholesterol, is the so-called bad cholesterol. This substance contributes to the development of heart disease by depositing cholesterol in the walls of the coronary arteries, narrowing them. On the other hand, *high-density lipoprotein* cholesterol, or HDL cholesterol, blocks the accumulation of LDL by transferring it away from the arteries.

Triglycerides are the chemical form in which most fat exists in the body. They are derived from fats eaten in food or manufactured in the body. Hormones regulate the release of triglycerides from fat tissue so they can meet the body's energy needs between meals.

Here is how total blood cholesterol levels stack up (cholesterol is measured in milligrams per deciliter of blood).

Total Blood Cholesterol

Desirable	200 mg/dl
Borderline high	200–239 mg/dl
High	240 mg/dl or higher

If your total cholesterol is over 200, you're not necessarily at risk. If it's high because your HDL cholesterol level is high, the total may be nothing to worry about; it's probably good, in fact. Women, particularly prior to menopause, are more likely to have these high HDL levels.

The following tables show what levels are healthy and not healthy for the three lipoproteins.

HDL Cholesterol Levels

Desirable   35 or greater (many doctors prefer 45 or higher)
Not desirable   Under 35

Somtimes a ratio instead of a number is used to explain the HDL cholesterol level; the total cholesterol number is divided by the HDL cholesterol level. For example, if you have a total cholesterol of 200 and an HDL cholesterol level of 50, the ratio would be stated as 4:1 (four to one). A desirable cholesterol ratio is below 5:1.

LDL Cholesterol Levels

Desirable	Under 130 mg/dl
Borderline to high	130–159 mg/dl
High	160 mg/dl or higher

Triglycerides

Normal	Less than 200 mg/dl
Borderline-high	200–400 mg/dl
High	400–1,000 mg/dl
Very high	1,000 mg/dl or higher

Currently these are the categories of cholesterol levels, but keep an eye on research, because this may very well change.

When the relationship between cholesterol and heart disease became evident, a national campaign was launched to "Know Your Cholesterol Level." But since nearly half of the people with heart disease have normal cholesterol levels, it's becoming more and more evident that this measurement is far too broad an indicator. In fact, it's been learned that there are many different cholesterol patterns—over a dozen have been identified so far—and it's not necessarily their components, but the way in which they are arranged, that determines their danger. Research is underway, but in the meantime here are some examples of the patterns that are garnering interest: Lipoprotein (a), LDL pattern A, and LDL pattern B.

Although it was initially assumed that all LDL cholesterol is harmful, some are more dangerous than others. For example, LDL pattern A so far seems to be one of the less dangerous forms of LDL cholesterol, because its larger, fluffier particles don't seem to have the talent for clogging up arteries that some of the other patterns do. For instance, the pattern called Lipoprotein (A), also known as Lp (a), appears to be double trouble; this pattern not only aids in the formation of heart attack-causing blood clots, it also contributes to atherosclerosis by leading to the overgrowth of smooth muscle tissue inside the coronary artery's walls.

Another deadly pattern is LDL pattern B. Studies thus far have identified it in one of every three men, and one of every five to six postmenopausal women. In this pattern, the particles are small, dense, and particularly effective in packing the arteries. In addition, people with this pattern also have less protective HDL cholesterol and higher triglycerides. So studies indicate that people with LDL pattern B have a threefold risk of heart disease, even if they have high HDL cholesterol and a low LDL level generally.

It's being learned that these different cholesterol patterns carry different treatment implications. For instance, some small studies indicate that a diet low in fat, while effective in people with LDL pattern B, may be less useful, possibly even harmful, for some people with LDL pattern A. This work is still in the research stages, but it eventually may explain why some people cannot lower their cholesterol levels despite diet and exercise and may also lead to cholesterol-fighting strategies that can be individually tailored. This is an exciting field, and before long a wider range of tests to uncover particular cholesterol patterns—and a larger variety of treatments—may be available. In the meantime, ask your doctor about these tests if you have a family medical history that puts you at high risk for heart disease, especially if you have a parent, brother, or sister who developed heart disease under the age of 45. If your doctor is unfamiliar with these tests, contact a well-known medical center with a top-notch cardiology department.

Homocysteine

In the past few years, attention has focused on *homocysteine*, an amino acid in the blood that, at abnormally high levels, is suspected of causing heart attacks. Although it isn't known how homocysteine may contribute to atherosclerosis, it's speculated that too much of this substance damages the inner lining of the coronary arteries and promotes blood clots.

Much remains unknown. For example, the level of high homocysteine varies between individuals, and it's not clear what level is dangerous. It's also unknown if reducing these levels to normal will prevent heart disease. Furthermore, the cause-and-effect relationship between homocysteine and heart disease has not yet been established, so it's not certain whether the problem is the homocysteine itself or the fact that a high level of it is a marker for a related factor that is actually the villain. For instance, people with high homocysteine levels have low levels of vitamin B_6 as well, and some think that the low levels of vitamin B_6 may be doing the harm.

Being Overweight

If you weigh 20 percent or more than your ideal body weight, it's long been known, you are at increased risk for heart disease. Being overweight in general is detrimental, but there is evidence that this effect is heightened depending on how that excess weight is distributed. If it has settled in your stomach, making you apple-shaped, you are worse off, in terms of health, than your pear-shaped friends.

Here's how to determine if you have a healthy waist-to-hip ratio. Take a tape measure and measure around your waist at the navel level (no cheating—don't pull in your stomach). Then measure your hips at their widest. Divide the waist measurement by the hip measurement for your waist-to-hip ratio. If you're a man, the ideal ratio is 0.95. For a woman it's 0.80.

A Sedentary Lifestyle

Being a couch potato is bad for the heart. In the past, being inactive has been associated with being overweight, but studies find that a sedentary lifestyle in itself is a major risk factor for heart disease. In addition, women who don't exercise are more likely to have abnormal cholesterol patterns, high blood pressure, and diabetes, all of which lay the groundwork for heart disease.

Stress

From all the discussion of the health hazards of stress in the media, you would think that it is the cause of nearly all heart attacks in women. But the impact of stress on the heart is not clearly understood. One of the reasons that stress is so difficult to study is that people react differently to it. Flo, for example, enjoys stepping up to the microphone; asked to say a few words after dinner, she is always at ease. But Barbara, asked to say a few words at a family dinner, couldn't wait for the occasion to be over. "My palms were sweating, I was all tense, I couldn't breathe," she recalled.

Still, evidence is mounting that emotional response—particularly anger and hostility—may contribute to heart disease, notes Rita Watson, M.P.H., an author living in New Haven, Connecticut, who writes and lectures about the health effects of stress.

"Everyone knows how stressful divorce, job loss, or a move to another part of the country can be. But the impact of less obvious stress-producing events often goes unrecognized. These more subtle stressors, such as an unfulfilling job, a rocky marriage, or just sitting in commuter traffic day in and day out can be damaging," she said.

When you're under stress, your body's autonomic nervous system responds by increasing production of such hormones as epinephrine, which increases your heart rate, pumps up your blood pressure, and speeds up your metabolism. This is known as the fight or flight response.

This cascade of hormones is thought to affect your heart in at least two ways. First, some researchers theorize that the hormonal increase you experience under stress keeps the LDL (bad) cholesterol circulating in your bloodstream longer, leading to heart disease.

Second, experts believe that people who are easily emotionally "aroused," that is, easily angered or made impatient, are vulnerable to hormone surges. In rare cases, it's believed, such surges can trigger a malfunction of the heart's electrical system, causing a heart attack or even death.

In looking at how stress may affect women's hearts in particular, another theory focuses on a woman's estrogen level. Since women usually develop heart disease after menopause, it is very likely that estrogen, the so-called female sex hormone, plays a key role in protecting the female heart. Some researchers, doing experiments with female monkeys, have found that when they are placed in subordinate positions to the dominant females, they produce less estrogen and tend to develop heart disease.

It's also been found that when they're under stress, women tend to smoke more and eat too much, habits that can raise the risk of heart disease as well.

It has long been believed that job stress can cause heart attacks in men, so that idea has been applied to women; thus, it's too often assumed that the reason women have high rates of heart disease is that, in some ways, this is a payback for having careers. "You work like a man, now you're having heart attacks like men" is the way this line of thinking goes.

This myth ignores the fact that heart disease in women is not new and so was not brought about by the feminist revolution. According to the American Heart Association's statistics, heart disease has been the leading killer of women since 1908.

There is, though, some evidence that certain types of work can be hazardous to the heart. The Framingham Heart Study, a large, three-generation study of heart disease risk factors that is still ongoing, found that women who were employed outside the home had lower death rates than those who were homemakers. However, researchers find this benefit does not extend to women in all types of jobs. Two groups of employed women who have higher rates of heart disease are those who work at low-level jobs where they have no autonomy, such as doing clerical work, and those who work rotating shifts. Although it isn't known exactly how shift work may impact heart health, it's theorized that the chronic disruption of the body's natural timing triggers the production of damaging stress-related hormones. Similar results have been found in studies of men who work rotating shifts.

Another related factor that may impact a woman's heart health is the multiple roles that modern women play. Today the vast majority of women work outside the home, either out of choice or economic necessity, but most also raise families. Often a woman's workday, unlike a man's, does not end when she leaves the office. A Swedish study, which has since been replicated in the United States, comparing male and female managers, found that at workday's end the stress-related hormones in the men's blood declined. The levels of stress-related hormones in the women's blood rose, an indication that they were not "winding down" but instead were gearing up for their homemaker demands.

Depression

Almost everyone feels sad or blue at one time or another. That kind of transient emotion is not the type considered a risk factor for heart disease. The kind of emotional state that may increase the risk of heart disease is clinical depression: the feeling of intense sadness that descends following a recent loss or sad event but is out of proportion to the event or lingers indefinitely. Or it may be persistent sadness that occurs for no reason at all. Exactly why depression increases the risk of heart disease is not known, but being depressed may produce hormonal changes that stimulate the body's autonomic nervous system, which raises blood pressure, constricts blood vessels, and increases heart rate. This may contribute to heart disease, some experts believe. If you are depressed, discuss it with your doctor; depression is a serious, but treatable, ailment in itself.

HOW TO REDUCE THE RISK OF HEART DISEASE

Quit Smoking

This is the healthiest thing you can do for your heart. Once you quit, your risk of suffering a heart attack immediately diminishes. Your risk is reduced by a third within 2 years, although it takes 10 to 14 years for all that added risk to disappear. For more information, see chapter 15.

Lose Weight

Throughout this book you'll see this recommendation. If you're seriously overweight, that can seem like a momentous task. However, research shows that even a modest weight loss—5 to 10 percent of body weight—can significantly lower heart disease risk. For tips on losing weight, see chapter 16.

Start Exercising

It's long been known that exercise lowers a man's risk of heart disease; over the past several years evidence has been mounting that this is true for women as well. Several studies have found that regular exercise can lower a woman's risk, in some cases by 40 percent or even more. This is true for women of all ages. Studies also find that the fitter the woman is, the lower her risk.

Exercise improves a woman's risk profile in several ways. For instance, a 1995 study at the American College of Cardiology found that the women who exercise the least have the worst cholesterol levels, glucose levels, and blood-pressure readings. These results improve with only modest exercise, such as taking a brisk 30 to 40-minute daily walk. In addition, exercise is a terrific stress reliever and mood enhancer. For more information, see chapter 17.

Consider Aspirin

If you are a middle-aged woman at average or high risk for a heart attack, a daily aspirin to prevent blood clots could be an excellent, low-cost treatment. There has been much publicity about the use of aspirin in men, but not in women, so it's not surprising that a 1997 study in the *Archives of Internal Medicine* found that women are less likely to take aspirin. The Nurses' Health Study found that low-dose aspirin reduced the risk of a first heart attack by about 30 percent. An Israeli study published in 1995 found a similar benefit. Aspirin, though, can have negative side effects for women who have bleeding problems or ulcers, so discuss it with your doctor before you begin taking it on a regular basis.

Consider Hormone Replacement Therapy

As noted earlier, women have a 10-to-15-year period of gender protection, and their rate of heart disease begins climbing only after menopause. An analysis of the many studies that have been done over the years shows that estrogen may decrease a woman's risk of heart disease by up to 50 percent. For more information, see chapter 18.

Estrogen is believed to have a multipronged beneficial effect on the heart. Research shows that estrogen favorably affects a woman's cholesterol pattern, making it less likely for heart attack–causing blood clots to form. There's also evidence that estrogen keeps a woman's coronary arteries more supple, protecting them from the stiffness that comes with age.

An important consideration in taking HRT is the increased risk of breast or uterine cancer. For more information, see chapter 18.

Reduce Your Stress

Reducing stress in your life can be more difficult than it sounds. But it pays off. In addition to possibly reducing the risk of heart disease, easing stress can also help women who find that they eat or smoke when they're under pressure. Here are some strategies.

Meditation

Meditation is a process in which one tries to achieve awareness without thought. Depending on your personality, there are two different types of meditation that might appeal to you. Transcendental Meditation (TM), which was popularized by the Maharishi Mahesh Yogi in the United States in the 1970s, teaches practitioners to focus on a single object, or a short phrase called a mantra. On the other hand, practitioners of "mindfulness" meditation learn to pay close attention to each moment. Mindfulness meditation, based on learning to live in the present, is an excellent way not only to reduce stress but also to eliminate unnecessary worrying.

Yoga

Relaxation, deep breathing, meditation, and stretching your body are all stress reducers. Yoga, a system of Hindu philosophy and religion, combines all three.

The form of yoga most familiar to Westerners is hatha yoga, in which the follower practices a series of poses, known as asanas, and uses a special breathing technique. These exercises maintain flexibility and teach physical and mental control.

In addition, yoga practitioners learn the same type of deep, abdominal breathing that is the foundation of many relaxation methods. They use breathing to help clear the mind and slow thoughts, both during asanas and in meditation.

Exercise

In addition to promoting good cardiovascular health, exercise is also an excellent stress reliever.

Consume Alcohol with Care

There is some evidence that alcohol—be it beer, wine, or liquor—may, when enjoyed in moderation, be good for the heart. For more information, see chapter 16.

HEART DISEASE WARNING SIGNS

Too often a heart attack is the first indication a woman has that something is wrong with her heart. But there are warning signs. If they are recognized and treated in time, that heart attack may be avoided.

Chest pain usually is considered a typical warning sign of heart disease—and, when it occurs more severely, for heart attacks. However, unaccountable fatigue and unusual shortness of breath, especially in women, can be warning signs as well.

Women do suffer from chest pain more often than men, and often it's not related to their hearts. Osteoarthritis in the neck, certain stomach problems, even simple gas—all these can cause pain in the chest. Sometimes it's impossible to tell heart-related chest pain from the non-heart–related variety. In this case, don't diagnose yourself; see your doctor.

What follows are descriptions of the two types of chest pain associated with heart disease.

Angina pectoris is the classic type of chest pain; it occurs when your heart muscle does not receive enough oxygen because of a narrowing in your coronary arteries, usually caused by atherosclerosis. It most often occurs during physical exertion. People who have it describe the feeling in their chest in various ways, including dull, aching, tingling, burning, tightness, squeezing, heaviness, constriction, or a sensation of pressure. They may feel anxious and unable to breathe. The pain may move around, often radiating from the middle of the chest, to the base of the neck or the left shoulder, down either the left or right arms, or into the jaw or sometimes the shoulder blade. The pain lasts at least a few minutes and is relieved by rest. Generally it occurs with exertion, doing activities in the cold, after a heavy meal, or under emotional stress.

Vasospastic angina, the second type of angina, may also be caused by the arteries of the heart going into spasm. This type is known by different names, including vasospastic angina, variant angina, or Printzmetal's angina, after the doctor who first described it. This type of angina results from blood being blocked as it flows to the heart muscle, not from a narrowing of the coronary arteries but because the coronary artery goes into spasm. Interestingly, although this type of angina is considered "atypical" for men, it may be more typical for women than the so-called classic angina pectoris. Remember that virtually all the knowledge about heart disease is based on research done on men.

With vasospastic angina, the quality and location of the chest pain is similar to that of regular angina pectoris, but typically it occurs when a person is at rest, sometimes in the early hours of the morning and sometimes repeatedly each night. The pain lasts longer, sometimes up to a half hour, and intensifies quickly. Vasospastic angina seems to affect mostly (but not only) women who are relatively young and heavy smokers. Sometimes episodes seem to be brought on with stress.

Beat Your Risk: Even if you've only begun experiencing it, the pain from either type of angina is a signal that something may be seriously wrong with your heart. Don't delay; call and talk to your doctor about it immediately.

HEART ATTACK WARNING SIGNS

Here are the typical signs of a heart attack. The warning signs in a woman can sometimes be more subtle, and include symptoms such as fatigue, nausea, and shortness of breath.

You may be having a heart attack if:

- The chest pain of heart attack comes on suddenly over a minute or two and builds in intensity.
- The pain occurs near the center of your chest.
- The pain lasts at least 20 minutes and is not relieved by rest or by changing position.
- The pain ranges from mild to severe and usually feels like tightness or heaviness.
- The pain radiates up into your jaw, your back, or down your left arm.

• You experience nausea, shortness of breath, or a sense of impending doom.

If you are experiencing possible cardiac symptoms, but your doctor does not take the possibility of heart disease seriously, be persistent. If you are brushed off, persist some more, or consider changing doctors.

Don't ignore the warning signs of heart disease or an impending heart attack. A heart attack, medically known as a *myocardial infarction* (MI), occurs when the blood flowing to your heart is cut off completely.

It is possible to suffer a silent heart attack, a symptomless heart attack that can go unnoticed but cause damage. These are believed to occur more often in women than in men.

Even when a woman is suffering symptoms, she may put off getting help, sometimes with tragic results. If you ignore heart attack symptoms, you are not only risking your life but also forfeiting the possibility that prompt emergency treatment could minimize the damage done to your heart. Clot busters, powerful drugs that can dissolve heart attack–causing clots, can reduce the damage caused by a heart attack or even prevent it. But these drugs are most effective only when administered within the first few hours after the heart attack begins.

Beat Your Risk: If you think you may be having a heart attack, do not attempt to drive yourself to the hospital. When you arrive at the emergency room, state that you believe you are having a heart attack and clearly relate your symptoms as specifically as possible; emergency workers do not take seriously a woman they deem "hysterical."

SCREENING FOR HEART DISEASE

One of the reasons heart disease in women is so serious is that it is often not diagnosed until a heart attack occurs. But there are effective screening tests to detect high blood pressure, diabetes, and abnormal cholesterol levels, three conditions that lead to heart disease. You should have your blood pressure monitored regularly. The guidelines for diabetes screening were given in the last chapter.

Cholesterol Screening

If you are over 20, you should have a cholesterol profile done to find out your ratio of the HDL (good) to the LDL (bad) cholesterol. If it's normal, you should be retested every five years. If it's borderline, a follow-up test every year or two is recommended. Triglyceride levels are usually measured when the total cholesterol level is elevated or when it is needed to compute LDL levels.

At the moment there is no agreement on whether additional cholesterol screening to determine other components, such as Lp (a) and LDL pattern B, is necessary. But, as noted earlier, if you suffered a heart attack under the age of 45, or if you have a parent or sibling who did, you should have these additional tests.

There is also no general agreement on homocysteine screening, but you should be tested if you have a family medical history of homocystinuria (an inherited condition that leads to high homocysteine levels) or if you're a young adult who has had a heart attack or symptoms of one. Again, check with your doctor for the latest status on this type of testing.

Tests for Heart Disease

Although there is screening for diseases that contribute to heart disease, a general screening test to detect it in women has proved elusive. If you are experiencing possible symptoms, there are diagnostic tests, but these are unsuitable as screening tools. Familiarize yourself with them, though, since they are the tests that will be used if you suspect you have heart disease.

The following are the most common tests, listed in order of how they would usually be administered in a nonemergency setting. The actual order in which they are done depends on a woman's individual case and her doctor's preference.

Electrocardiogram (ECG or EKG)

An *electrocardiogram* displays the electrical impulses your heart produces as it beats. A healthy heart produces a predictable pattern. But, although changes in the pattern may alert your doctor to heart disease or even a heart attack, a normal tracing pattern does not rule it out.

Exercise Stress Test

Commonly referred to as a *stress test*, the purpose of an exercise stress test is to evaluate the way your heart responds to the physical stress of exercise—walking and jogging on a treadmill or pedaling a stationary bicycle. Before the test begins, leads are attached to your chest so that changes in your heartbeat can be measured. If you have arthritis or some other physical problem that inhibits you from exercising, you'll be given a drug called dobutamine, which mimics the effects of exercise.

Although this test can provide valuable information about the heart, it is too inaccurate to be used as a screening test. This is because an estimated 15 to 40 percent of such tests mistakenly diagnose heart disease. This occurs especially in women because a healthy woman's heartbeat, when depicted graphically, can display changes characteristic of a woman with heart disease. Precisely why this occurs is not known, but it may relate to the fact that women's bodies respond differently to exercise than men's or to a woman's fluctuating hormone levels. However, a stress test can accurately be used to rule out heart disease.

Because of these drawbacks, two other methods are used to improve the exercise stress test's accuracy, as follows.

Myocardial Perfusion Scan

This combination of an exercise stress test and a nuclear scanning procedure used to be referred to as a thallium stress test since thallium was the imaging agent employed, but now other imaging substances are used as well. This type of test is more accurate because instead of just relying on a graphic depiction of your heartbeat, it also produces images of your heart.

Exercise Echocardiography

This procedure combines the exercise stress test with *echocardiography*, which produces ultrasound pictures of the heart. The heart is evaluated with ultrasound before and after an exercise stress test. The images of the heart are then evaluated to determine if it is receiving an adequate blood supply.

Cardiac Catheterization

This is considered the gold standard of cardiac diagnostic testing, but because, as an invasive procedure, it does carry a small degree of risk, it is generally done not only to confirm a diagnosis of heart disease but also to determine the need and to map plans for such procedures as cardiac bypass surgery or coronary angioplasty.

For this procedure you are awake but sedated. A thin catheter is inserted into a blood vessel, usually an artery in the leg or arm, and passed through it into the heart. Dye is injected to make the coronary arteries visible on X rays.

A Word about Testing

Over the years doctors have amassed an arsenal of sophisticated diagnostic tools, and more are on the horizon. It's easy for a doctor to be seduced by this wealth of fancy instrumentation. Valuable as these tests are, they are enhanced by the information you give your doctor when you know your family's medical history and your risk factors for heart disease.

THE BOTTOM LINE

Heart attack is the biggest killer of women, but you don't have to be a victim. Knowing your risk factors and taking advantage of the available screening tests, keeping up with the latest advances, such as those dealing with cholesterol patterns, and making lifestyle changes, such as quitting smoking, losing weight, and regularly exercising, can combine to help you conquer the odds.

Rate Your Risk: Heart Disease

Put a check mark after each answer. Answer all questions. Then consult the scoring key to compute your score.

	Score	
Family History	(+ column)	(− column)

1. Was your father or brother diagnosed with heart disease or did either suffer a heart attack? _____ _____

   Yes_____ +1   No _____ 0

2. If yes, at what age did this occur? _____ _____

   Before age 39   _____+3

   40–54   _____+2

   55–64   _____+1

   After 65   _____0

3. Has your mother or a sister been diagnosed with heart disease or did either suffer a heart attack? _____ _____

   Yes_____ +1   No _____ 0

4. If yes, at what age did this occur? _____ _____

   Before age 49   _____+3

   50–64   _____+2

   65–74   _____+1

   After 75   _____0

5. What is your race? _____ _____

   African-American   +5

   White or other   +3

Personal History/Habits

6. What is your age? _____ _____

   20–39   _____0

   40–54   _____+2

   Over 55   _____+3

7. If you are in or past menopause, are   _____ _____
   you on hormone replacement therapy?
   Yes_____   −3
   No_____   0

8. Do you weigh 20 pounds or more than   _____ _____
   you should?
   Yes_____   +2
   No_____   0

9. Do you take medication to lower your   _____ _____
   blood pressure?
   Yes_____   +4
   No_____   0

10. Have you been told your cholesterol   _____ _____
    level is too high?
    Yes_____   +3
    No_____   0

11. Do you have diabetes?   _____ _____
    Yes_____   +3
    No_____   0

12. Do you smoke?   _____ _____
    Yes_____   +3
    No_____   0

13. Do you smoke and take oral   _____ _____
    contraceptives?
    Yes_____   +5
    No_____   0

14. Are you generally inactive, that is,   _____ _____
    you spend most of your leisure time
    reading or watching TV?
    Yes_____   +2
    No_____   0

15. Do you exercise at least 30 minutes a
    day 3 days a week or more?
    Yes_____   −1
    No_____   0
       Subtotal   _____
       Risk Factor   +5
       (add in only if you answered
       yes to all or either #12 or 13)
       Final Score   _____

How to Score

1. Fill in the numbers in the columns at the far right.
2. Subtotal your score from the plus and minus columns.
3. Add the +5 if you answered yes to particular risk factors.
4. Compute your final score.
5. Compare your score to the Risk Factor Scoring Chart.

Heart Disease Risk Factor Scoring Chart

9 or below   Lowest risk

10 to 18   Low to moderate

19 to 27   Moderate to high

Above 28   Highest risk

CHAPTER 13

OSTEOPOROSIS

IMAGINE THAT YOUR FAMILIAR SURROUNDINGS suddenly become dangerous. A misstep could fracture your ankle. Reaching for a book could shatter a wrist. Just rolling over in bed could fracture the vertebrae in your spine.

This nightmare is real for the victims of osteoporosis. Just ask Sandy. Now 62, she was diagnosed with osteoporosis fifteen years ago. At first she was unconcerned. Her mother had osteoporosis, and it hadn't affected her. But Sandy's disease was more severe. A few years ago, at a concert in the park, she tripped over the roots of an old tree. "That was the beginning of it all," she recalls. Since then, she's suffered 32 fractures.

"I've sustained some of the fractures during three falls, but most are what is called 'voluntary fractures.' This means they just happen; a bone snaps if I bend over or reach across the sink," she says. She sustained two broken bones from as simple a task as the day she ironed using spray starch. Some of the spray got onto the floor and made it as slippery as an ice-skating rink. "I went flying and broke two bones," she recalls ruefully.

She has spent months in bed, weeks in a wheelchair. Sometimes she only needs a cane. She dreads the winter, which brings with it the ice that makes it too dangerous for her to venture outside, imprisoning her in her apartment.

WHAT IS OSTEOPOROSIS?

Osteoporosis is a progressive disease in which the bones become brittle and fracture easily. Its effects are most apparent in the elderly, but it can affect middle-aged women. Even if it doesn't, the seeds for osteoporosis in later life are sown when women are much younger. By taking measures then, you can prevent this disease that can turn your later years into a nightmare of wheelchairs and nursing homes.

Osteoporosis is a progressive decrease in the density of the bones that weakens them and makes them easy to fracture. The bones become porous, the characteristic that gives this disease its name, and honeycombed with holes. Sometimes it doesn't even take a fall to splinter them; the bones grow so weak they simply shatter.

Of the 25 million Americans afflicted with osteoporosis, the vast majority are women. Every year this disease causes an estimated 1.3 million fractures, including 500,000 spinal crush fractures, 250,000 hip fractures, and 200,00 wrist fractures. Shoulder, shin, and pelvic fractures make up the remainder.

All of these osteoporosis-caused fractures have three things in common:

- They occur mostly in people over the age of 35.
- They occur mostly in women.
- They occur in the absence of severe injury. In fact, a clue to osteoporosis is a fracture that is caused by a seemingly minor mishap, such as a mild turn that breaks an ankle or a slight fall that fractures a wrist.

The Hip Fracture

Fran was known for her independent spirit. Graduating Phi Beta Kappa from an Ivy League school in the days when girls rarely went to college, she went on to become a teacher. Retirement didn't stop her; well into her seventies, she drove her friends to movies and concerts. Most of all she enjoyed singing with a group that performed for nursing home patients.

Standing on the curb one winter day, she tumbled to the ground. Was it a slip on the ice, or did her bone shatter of its own accord? She doesn't know. In any case, from that day on, her life was changed. Now she can barely manage to go from her bed to sit in the living room without help. No more driving, no last-minute excursions to the store, no singing group. The independent life she relished is gone.

The hip fracture is the most dreaded result of osteoporosis, and with good reason. Women over the age of 75 suffer hip fractures twice as often as men. Of those who suffer this fracture, 5 to 20 percent die eventually of complications from being bedridden, including blood clots and pneumonia. About half will never walk, or won't walk as well. Only the minority—20 percent—regain their previous abilities.

Osteoporosis exacts another steep price as well. If taking only a short walk can cause you a fracture, it's not surprising if you become housebound. Osteoporosis alters a woman's appearance as she shrinks in height, her clothes no longer fit, and, eventually, what used to be known as a *dowager's hump* can form.

But osteoporosis truly is one of those diseases where an ounce of prevention is worth a pound of cure. Unfortunately, prevention is rarely emphasized; attention is paid only after fractures begin occurring, if then. These fractures are thought of only as the inevitable effect of old age, not only by women but too often by their doctors. Nowadays, with more ways to prevent osteoporosis, this view must change.

All About Bone

Our skeletons are made up of 206 bones. Although we usually think of our bones as being rock solid, they are actually composed of living tissue, which is formed into hydroxyapatite. Calcium is the principal ingredient of this hard, cementlike substance. But calcium is used not only to keep the skeleton strong. For our body to work properly, there needs to be enough calcium in our bloodstream, because calcium helps transmit signals from our nerves to our muscles. Therefore, it keeps our heart beating, our muscles contracting, and our blood pressure stable. If this calcium level drops below a critical level, it is taken from the bones. To provide this calcium, bone is constantly being built, a process called *formation*, and being broken down, which is called *resorption*. Together, this complex process is called *bone remodeling*, and it occurs throughout our life. If formation outpaces resorption, bone density increases; if bone is broken down and not replaced, bone loss occurs.

Normally this constant remodeling process causes no problems; the cavities created in the bone are filled in with new tissue and remain strong. But if bone loss occurs over time, osteoporosis results. Eventually, the bones become brittle, pockmarked by holes, and fractures result.

Three terms are used throughout this chapter to discuss the components of your bones:

Bone mineral content—the total amount of calcium in your bones
Bone mass—the total amount of calcium plus all the other minerals in your bones
Bone density—the bone mineral content in relation to the width of your bones

FACTORS THAT INCREASE YOUR RISK OF OSTEOPOROSIS

Being Female

Osteoporosis occurs overwhelmingly more often in women than in men. This is because a woman's bones are lighter and less dense to begin with, so they fracture more easily.

Growing Older

As we age, our ability to make new bone diminishes and our risk of osteoporosis rises. In the past osteoporosis was commonly thought of as a "little old lady" ailment, and there is some truth to that. For instance, if you're 50, you have a 15 percent risk of suffering a hip fracture over your entire lifetime. By the time you reach 80, you bear that same 15 percent hip-fracture risk during the nine remaining years of your life expectancy.

However, you should start thinking about osteoporosis when you're 50—or even earlier—as opposed to 80! Although the effects of osteoporosis are seen most sharply in the elderly, if you're at particular risk for it, it can afflict you at a much younger age. Furthermore, the choices you make when you're younger can help prevent osteoporosis or contribute to it.

Race

White and Asian women are at highest risk for osteoporosis. Because the bones of African-American women are denser, osteoporosis is less common; however, as they age, their risk of osteoporosis and hip fracture does increase. Between 80 to 95 percent of fractures in African-American women over the age of 64 are due to osteoporosis; as they age, their risk of hip fracture doubles approximately every seven years. Furthermore, certain diseases more prevalent among African-Americans, such as sickle-cell anemia, are linked to osteoporosis.

Although Latina women are usually considered at less risk for osteoporosis than white or Asian women, this problem should not be ignored. Like white and Asian women, they tend to consume less calcium than they need to maintain strong bones.

Family Medical History

Your risk of osteoporosis is greater if it runs in your family. Does it run in yours? To figure this out, you may only need to take a good look at your relatives, notes Karl Insogna, M.D., director of the Yale Bone Center at the Yale University School of Medicine.

"A lot of my women come to the center after they've encountered an older relative they haven't seen for a while. A woman may tell me, 'I came to see you because I recently saw my aunt, and she's so hunched over. I don't want this happening to me.'"

Here are red flags to consider when leafing through the family photo album. Have your relatives:

- Lost height as they aged?
- Had curvature of the spine?
- Suffered fractures as they've grown older, particularly from falls or accidents that were relatively minor?

If you resemble in appearance your relatives with these characteristics, this is a clue that you may have inherited a genetic tendency for this disease as well.

Being Postmenopausal

Although you usually think of estrogen in connection with your reproductive system, it is an essential part of the bone-remodeling process. Therefore, your risk of osteoporosis increases when you reach menopause and your estrogen level declines. An estimated 75 percent of spinal fractures and up to 65 percent of hip fractures are due to this postmenopausal bone loss. In fact, "the scope of the osteoporosis problem in postmenopausal women is staggering," writes Dr. Robert Lindsay, professor of clinical medicine at Columbia University and president of the National Osteoporosis Foundation.

Not all loss of bone is due to menopause; it's believed that both men and women begin to lose bone mass from the spine beginning in their twenties. But a woman's rate of bone loss accelerates sharply after menopause for up to about eight years, and then it diminishes, although it can continue at a rate of up to 5 percent a year in some women.

These figures don't mean that all such women develop osteoporosis. Although all women lose estrogen at menopause, only some develop osteoporosis. "Some women are 'bone savers' and some are 'bone losers,' and we don't know why," says Dr. Lila Wallis, clinical professor of medicine at Cornell University Medical College.

Having Premature Menopause

If you're in menopause because of artificial means, such as having had your ovaries removed or due to chemotherapy or radiation, you could develop osteoporosis. When you go through menopause naturally, your estrogen level declines gradually, and your body still manufactures a small amount of it even after your periods stop. However, if most of your estrogen production suddenly ceases, your bone loss declines even more quickly.

Beat Your Risk: In the past, a woman's ovaries were routinely removed during hysterectomy. If you are going to undergo a hysterectomy, and there is no medical necessity to remove your ovaries, ask that they be retained. The estrogen they will continue to produce until menopause will protect you not only from osteoporosis but also from heart disease.

Being Slender and Small-Boned

Slender, small-boned women are more prone to osteoporosis than larger women, because they have less bone to begin with. How do you know if you're small-boned? A tip-off is if your shoe size is 6½ or smaller. Women who are heavier are also at less risk because they tend to retain more estrogen after menopause. Furthermore, to carry the extra weight, their bones remain stronger. But this isn't a reason to put on extra pounds; too much excess weight causes arthritis and joint problems.

Certain Medical Disorders

Several medical conditions can raise the risk of osteoporosis. They are:

Diabetes

Type I diabetes, formerly known as juvenile diabetes, can increase the risk, especially if it's been poorly controlled or you've been on large doses of insulin. This is not to be confused with Type II, or adult-onset, diabetes, which was discussed earlier and is the most common form of diabetes. Type II diabetes does not raise osteoporosis risk.

Menstrual Irregularities

Women whose periods cease due to eating disorders or excessive exercise are at increased risk of osteoporosis. Although the trend among women to be more active is to be applauded, young athletes who are so thin they stop menstruating are very vulnerable as well. In fact, the spinal density in some female athletes in their twenties has been found to resemble that of women in their seventies and eighties. Women who have irregular menstrual periods or whose periods cease for reasons such as hormone imbalances are also at increased risk for osteoporosis. If you have irregular periods, see your doctor.

Certain Endocrine Disorders

These hormonal disorders are associated with bone loss:

Hyperparathyroidism: the excessive secretion of parathyroid hormone, which helps regulate blood calcium levels.

Hyperthyroidism: overactivity of the thyroid gland, which can lead to an accelerated rate of bone breakdown.

Hyperprolactinemia: a condition characterized by an increased blood level of prolactin, the hormone involved in breast milk production.

Cushing's syndrome: a disorder in which the adrenal glands produce too much of the hormone cortisol, leading to excessive bone loss.

By the way, *scoliosis*, an abnormal curvature of the spine, which occurs predominantly in girls, may also increase the risk of osteoporosis later in life.

The Typical American Diet

America is among the countries with the highest rates of osteoporosis in the world. Unfortunately, our salty, protein-rich diet is probably a chief reason.

As noted earlier, our bones store calcium, breaking it down for use by our cells. As this store of calcium is depleted, more and more bone is broken down to compensate. This contributes to osteoporosis.

Calcium is not a mineral that is easily absorbed or retained in the body. The first problem is getting enough calcium from the food we eat. Although calcium is contained in many foods, including dairy products, eating enough can be difficult, especially for women who diet too stringently.

But this isn't the only impediment. Calcium is very easily depleted, and some of the foods we eat have this effect. Here are the chief culprits:

- Sodium: The more salt you consume, the more calcium you excrete in your urine. Salt is widely found in the foods we enjoy. It is used in processed foods both as a preservative and a flavor enhancer. Sometimes you don't even realize it. Salt is obviously an ingredient in potato chips, but what about corn flakes? They may contain even more salt.
- Protein: Most of us were raised to look for protein as a major ingredient in our meals. But the problem is that although our bodies need some protein, most of us tend to eat too much of it. In a country that "super sizes" its fast-food hamburgers, this can be a major problem.
- Fiber: Although this is a very healthful substance, there is one down side; fiber can rob the body's store of calcium.
- Alcohol: Indulging in alcoholic beverages decreases the calcium in your body.
- Caffeine: Caffeine blocks the absorption of calcium.

You can compensate for some of this calcium loss by eating more wisely, as discussed in chapter 16. In addition, the government now recommends that all women take calcium supplements (discussed later in this chapter).

Inactivity

If you become less physically active as you age (and most women do), your bone density declines so gradually that you don't even notice it. Why is this? The action of pulling on bones strengthens them, increasing bone density. This is demonstrated by the amount of bone lost if you're bedridden. Astronauts once sustained bone loss from being weightless, and now exercise that strengthens bones is part of the regimen when women and men are sent into space.

Smoking

Cigarette smoking was first identified as a risk factor for osteoporosis more than 20 years ago. One key reason is that the anti-estrogen effect of tobacco smoke interferes with the building of strong bone. Also, some studies indicate smokers absorb calcium less effectively. Bone thinning from smoking occurs not only in older women who are more at risk for osteoporosis but in young female smokers. So at a time in their life when these young women should be building bone, they jeopardize it by smoking.

Drug-Induced Osteoporosis

Last year Barbara underwent a bone-density test. Her doctor had recommended it because for years she's had to rely on a steroids to stave off bouts of potentially life-threatening asthma. "I was shocked to find out that, even though I was only in my early fifties, I had signs of osteoporosis," Barbara says.

Drug-induced osteoporosis is a very important risk factor in women because they are more prone to many of the ailments these medications are prescribed for. This is especially true for *corticosteroids*, also known as *steroids*, which are given on a long-term basis for numerous ailments, including severe asthma, rheumatoid arthritis, ulcerative colitis, multiple sclerosis, and some blood and kidney diseases. While using these drugs for short periods isn't considered harmful, long-term use, especially at high dosages, is. It's estimated that fractures occur in one-third of the cases of drug-induced osteoporosis. This is because steroids are believed to adversely affect bone-forming cells; fewer are born, and they die prematurely. Weakened bones and fractures are the results, particularly in the hips and the spine. Age is not a factor; even children can be affected. In some cases the damage is so severe the person ends up in a wheelchair.

Other drugs that can weaken your bones are:

• *Thyroid hormone*—many women take this to speed up their sluggish thyroid glands. Taking too high an amount can cause osteoporosis.

• Heparin—used to prevent blood clots

• Anticonvulsants—such as phenytoin (Luminal) and phenobarbital (Dilantin), used to treat seizures

• Insulin—used to treat diabetes

• Diuretics—given to people with high blood pressure; some types can exacerbate the loss of calcium in the urine

• Gonadotropin-releasing hormone (GnRH)—the synthetic hormones used to treat gynecological problems, including endometriosis and uterine fibroids.

The adverse effects of these drugs depend on the dosage and length of time they are used. Sometimes doctors are unaware of the serious osteoporosis-causing effects of some of these drugs. Bring up this concern. Talk about possible alternatives. If this isn't possible, take steps to minimize bone loss through diet and exercise, calcium supplements and, if necessary, hormone or drug treatment (discussed later).

Beat Your Risk: *Although most of the osteoporosis-inducing drugs are given by prescription only, over-the-counter antacids that contain aluminum can also lead to calcium loss. If you're using such an antacid (Di-Gel, Gelusil, Maalox, and Mylanta are just a few), try to cut back and switch to ones that contain calcium, like Tums or Rolaids, which are actually used as calcium supplements.*

HOW TO REDUCE THE RISK OF OSTEOPOROSIS

Replenish Your Calcium Every Day

As noted, your body requires a constant supply of calcium to live; if the supply isn't maintained, calcium is taken from the bones. So you need to replenish your store of calcium every day, whether you're at risk for osteoporosis or not. It's now recommended that all women eat a diet that meets certain requirements for calcium. Here are the government's recommendations:

- 1,000 milligrams daily for premenopausal women between the ages of 25 and 49, or postmenopausal women ages 50 to 64 currently taking estrogen
- 1,500 milligrams daily for postmenopausal women ages 50 to 64 who are not taking estrogen and for all women over the age of 65

Although calcium is a difficult mineral for the body to absorb, you should get some of your daily requirements from the foods you eat. Sources include dairy products, including the low-fat type, salmon, sardines, and some bread and grain products. Broccoli, collard greens, and kale are all rich in calcium.

Since most women don't get enough calcium, supplements are recommended. In addition, you should make certain you're getting enough vitamin D, the "sunshine" vitamin that is absorbed through your skin. Recently it's been learned that adults may not get enough vitamin D, so a supplement may be warranted. Some calcium supplements also offer vitamin D. For more information, see chapter 16.

Exercise

The more stress you put on bone, the more the bone forms. That's physical, not emotional stress. Pulling on your muscles and bones strengthens them.

Which type of exercise is best? With osteoporosis the term to remember is "weight-bearing exercise." This means your body works against gravity, as compared with swimming, when you're buffered by the water.

"The best exercise for stress on bone is nice, brisk walking, swinging your arms. It's been shown that even with the most complicated equipment, nothing is better than walking," Lila E. Nachtigall, M.D., director of the Women's Wellness Division of Gynecology at the New York University School of Medicine in New York City said at a conference sponsored by the American Medical Women's Association in 1993.

For more bone-strengthening tips, see chapter 17.

Beat Your Risk: *Body-strengthening exercise is also important for women with osteoporosis. However, if you have osteoporosis, your fracture risk is high, so you should embark on a program that is designed by an exercise specialist and approved by your doctor.*

Quit Smoking

Although research indicates that smoking diminishes bone density, studies find that quitting, even later in life, can help minimize this loss.

Consider Preventative Treatments

Just a few years ago, the only preventive treatment for osteoporosis was estrogen. Now there is an increasing number of hormonal and nonhormonal treatments, and more are on the way. So if you are at significantly high risk for this disease, if you're already showing signs of it, or if you cannot take estrogen, you now have a much broader choice.

Hormone Replacement Therapy

Because estrogen is so important in the building and maintaining of bone, *estrogen replacement therapy* (ERT) has become a popular means of preventing osteoporosis. Numerous studies have found that women who take hormones, whether pure estrogen (ERT) or the combination of estrogen and progesterone (HRT), get stronger bones. In addition, raloxifen (Evista), the first of the so-called designer hormones, and a low-dose estrogen known as Estratab have been approved for the prevention of osteoporosis. For more information see chapter 18.

Nonhormonal Drugs

There are some women who shouldn't, or may be reluctant, to take even lower-dose and designer hormones. Because of this, non-hormonal osteoporosis preventatives are being developed.

Alendronate (Fosamax), a nonhormonal drug used to both prevent and treat osteoporosis, stops bone loss, increases density, and reduces fracture risks. Some effects are uncommon but may include irritation of the esophagus, abdominal or muscle and bone pain, nausea, and heartburn. As with estrogen, alendronate must be taken indefinitely to maintain its protective effect; once it is discontinued, bone loss resumes. Therefore, although Fosamax is an option for women who are at high risk for osteoporosis, its long-term effects are unknown. So if you decide to take it, stay aware of research findings.

Beat Your Risk: *Even if you went through menopause years ago, it's never too late to begin these therapies. You can't regain bone you lost, but you can increase your bone mass, reducing the risk of fractures.*

SCREENING FOR OSTEOPOROSIS

Because osteoporosis occurs without causing symptoms, it is usually not diagnosed until a fractures is suffered. Obviously, that's too late for prevention, so this is where screening comes in. As the baby boomer population ages, awareness of osteoporosis grows, and preventative treatments are developed, interest in screening is growing, and low-cost and even free screening is being offered.

Dr. Lindsay advocates much wider use of bone-density screening. It can predict osteoporotic fractures better than cholesterol levels for heart attacks, yet it is underutilized, he contends. On the other hand, the National Women's Health Network, a Washington, D.C.-based advocacy group, contends that widespread screening of post-menopausal women will result in too many of them deciding to take hormones or other preventative drugs. In addition, bone-density measurements have been obtained from white women and may not be as accurate in evaluating fracture risk in blacks and other minorities, the organization contends.

When deciding whether to undergo screening, begin by evaluating your risk factors. Bear in mind, though, that these predictors are not guarantees, and a woman can develop osteoporosis even in the absence of risk factors.

It remains to be determined whether the benefits of bone-density testing make it worthwhile for all postmenopausal women. Right now there are also no universally accepted guidelines of who should be screened; however, in 1998 Medicare was ordered to pay for screening for women in the following groups. Private insurers often follow Medicare's lead, so these categories will probably become standard.

- Women who are estrogen-deficient because their ovaries have been removed or postmenopausal women not taking estrogen-replacement therapy
- Women who have suffered vertebral fractures
- Women who are taking osteoporosis-inducing drugs on a long-term basis
- Women who have primary hyperparathyroidism, a condition that results in the excessive release of calcium from the bones

You should also consider screening if you have spinal abnormalities, if you have a strong family medical history of osteoporosis, or if you have other reasons to suspect you may be developing it—for instance if you surprisingly sustain a fracture from a non-severe accident.

When should you be screened, and how often? Again, there are no firm guidelines, but the recently enacted Medicare provision calls for rescreening every two years. If you're on osteoporosis-inducing drugs, you should discuss more frequent testing with your doctor.

If you're approaching menopause but are at low or average risk for osteoporosis, or you've decided to go on hormone replacement therapy anyway, you may decide against screening. But as the years pass, don't forget your bones; at some point have your bone density checked, perhaps at a landmark like your fiftieth birthday; then have it done every few years afterward. Should your risk factor situation change and, say, you become markedly less active, take this into consideration and have the test done sooner rather than waiting.

THE SCREENING TESTS

Conventional X rays are not used to screen for osteoporosis because they don't reveal a decline in bone mass until 30 percent has been lost. Because of this, a special type of bone imaging, known as *densitometry*, was developed. Bone-density measurement can detect bone loss before a fracture occurs as well as predict the likelihood of future fractures.

Currently, a bone imaging test known as *dual energy X-ray absorptiometry*, or DEXA, is the most popular and comprehensive. It is a simple, painless, and risk-free test that emits less radiation than a set of dental X rays. You lie down on a table while a special X ray camera passes over you, registering an image of the bone mass at the sites where osteoporotic bone loss occurs, including the hip and the spine. The machine compares the images to that of the normal bone density in a 35-year-old woman who is at peak bone mass. For every 10 percent decrease in bone density, the risk of fracture doubles.

Currently, DEXA is considered the most thorough form of bone imaging, because it measures the sites where osteoporosis is most likely to occur. The test, which takes less than a half hour, usually costs from about $150 to 200.

The SXA, or pDEXA, Test

Single X ray absorptiometry is a procedure which provides an image of the bone density in the forearm or heel. This test, known also as *peripheral densitometry*, or pDEXA, is done with a portable machine and is faster and cheaper than the DEXA procedures, so it can be done in the workplace or a shopping mall. The test measures bone density only at a single site, usually the wrist or the hip, and cannot accurately measure bones deeper in the body, including the hip or the spinal vertebrae. When free or low-cost screenings are offered, this is usually the type done.

Other bone-density testing procedures are on the horizon. These newer methods include an ultrasound test, which uses sound waves instead of radiation to measure bone density in the heel. Approved in 1998, it is designed to make screening more available and lower in cost than DEXA, but like the SXA procedure, it is not as comprehensive.

If you have a less comprehensive test done, don't depend on it to provide you with a complete picture of the state of your bones. Instead, consider it a prescreening test; if the results show you have low or lower than average bone density, have a DEXA test done.

Blood and Urine Tests

Several types of special urine and blood tests measure the rate of bone remodeling. These tests can show a high rate of bone turnover, which can be a sign of rapid bone loss. However, rates of bone turnover, like metabolism, vary from one person to another; a rate that signifies bone loss in one person may not for another.

These tests are appropriate when used in addition to bone-density screening or, if you're being treated for osteoporosis, to evaluate the medication's effect. However, these tests are sometimes promoted as a low-cost way to screen for osteoporosis, and they don't provide enough information to take the place of bone-density testing.

Screening Safeguards

If you decide to have your bone density measured, bear in mind that this type of screening is in its infancy, compared to, for example, mammography. Therefore, there are really no safeguards in place to make certain you get an accurate test result. The tests are simple to do but do require knowledge and skill to arrive at an accurate interpretation. So have your screening performed at a hospital or medical center or in the office of a doctor you trust. Ask if the technician performing the test is certified by the machine's manufacturer. If you're having a DEXA test done, make certain the technician is certified by the International Society of Clinical Densitometry.

THE WARNING SIGNS OF OSTEOPOROSIS

Studies show that six in ten people think that osteoporosis has warning signs. This is false. Just as people with high blood pressure may be unaware of it until they suffer a stroke, people with osteoporosis are often unaware of it until they suffer a fracture. A diagnosis of osteoporosis may come as a surprise to a woman who thinks she simply fractured a bone.

If you sustain a fracture due to a fall that should have produced only a very minor injury, that may be an important tip-off. For instance, breaking your wrist in a skiing accident is probably indicative of nothing but bad luck, but if the bone broke when you only slightly hit your wrist, this may indicate brittleness.

Another clue to osteoporosis may be gum disease and tooth loss. Researchers are investigating the relationship between bone loss density and tooth loss and gum disease, known also as *periodontitis*. If this research holds up, a routine dental X ray may eventually be used to screen for osteoporosis.

Beat Your Risk: *Don't mistake the warning signs of osteoarthritis for osteoporosis. Osteoarthritis, known commonly as arthritis, is a disease of the joints characterized by degeneration of the cartilage that leads to pain, swelling, and stiffness. Women often mistakenly think that these are also the warning signs of osteoporosis as well, so when they don't have these symptoms they assume nothing is amiss. The problem is, they might be wrong.*

Rate Your Risk: Osteoporosis

Put a check mark after each answer. Answer all questions. Then consult the scoring key to compute your score.

	Score	
	(+ column)	(– column)

Family History

1. Have any members of your close family _____ _____
   (grandmother, mother, sisters, aunts)
   developed osteoporosis?
   Yes_____ +1   No _____ 0

Personal History/Habits

2. What is your age?   _____ _____
   20–39   _____0
   40–54   _____+2
   Over 55   _____+3

3. What is your race?   _____ _____
   White   +3
   Asian   +3
   African-American   –1
   Other   0

4. Are you considered underweight or   _____ _____
   very slender?
   Yes_____ +2   No_____ 0

5. Do you wear a size 6 ½ shoe or smaller   _____ _____
   Yes_____ +2   No_____ 0

6. Are you in or past menopause   _____ _____
   Yes_____ +2   No_____ 0

7. If you are in menopause, did you   _____ _____
   experience it before the age of 40 due
   to the removal of your ovaries,
   chemotherapy, or radiation?
   Yes_____ +3   No_____ 0

8. If yes, do you take hormone _____ _____
   replacement therapy?
   Yes_____   –3   No_____   0

9. As you've grown older, has your height _____ _____
   decreased?
   Yes_____   +2   No_____   0

10. Have you ever been diagnosed with _____ _____
    any of these conditions?
    Hyperparathyroidism   +1
    Hyperprolactinemia   +1
    Liver disease   +1
    Hyperthyroidism   +1
    Cushing's Syndrome   +1

11. Have you been taking thyroid _____ _____
    medication or cortisone-like drugs
    for asthma, arthritis, or cancer on a
    prolonged basis?
    Yes_____   +3   No_____   0

12. Have you ever dieted excessively or _____ _____
    had an eating disorder?
    Yes_____   +1   No_____   0

13. Are you lactose intolerant? _____ _____
    Yes_____   +1   No_____   0

14. Do you eat a diet low in calcium or _____ _____
    dairy products?
    Yes_____   +1   No_____   0

15. Do you smoke? _____ _____ _____
    Yes_____   +1   No_____   0

16. Do you take calcium supplements _____ _____
    daily?
    Yes_____   –1   No_____   0

17. Do you exercise?   _____ _____

    Yes_____ −1   No_____ +1

18. If yes, do you perform strength-training_____ _____

    or weight-bearing exercise at least

    three days a week?

    Yes_____ −1   No_____ +1

19. Have you ever suffered a fracture for   _____ _____

    a very slight injury or no known cause?

    Yes_____ +2   No_____ 0

    Subtotal   _____

    Risk Factor   +5

    Final Score   _____

How to Score

1. Fill in the numbers in the columns at the far right.

2. Subtotal your score from the plus and minus columns.

3. Add the +5 if you answered yes to particular risk factors.

4. Compute your final score.

5. Compare your score to the Risk Factor Scoring Chart.

Osteoporosis Risk Factor Scoring Chart

10 or below   Lowest risk

11 to 20   Low to moderate

21 to 30   Moderate to high

Above 31   Highest risk

STROKE

THREE TIMES A WEEK, Emily gamely kicks up her heels in her aerobics class. She doesn't kick as high as many. But that she can do some steps, keep time to the beat, and perform at least some of the dance routines is a tribute to her persistence. Two years ago, at the age of 53, Emily suffered a stroke. It's commonly believed that strokes happen only to the elderly. Emily once thought that too. She doesn't anymore.

THE STROKE TOLL

About 500,000 Americans suffer a stroke every year, and slightly over half of them are women. An estimated 87,000 women die from it every year, the American Heart Association says.

"Stroke kills twice as many women as breast cancer. Stroke is the third cause of death for women in the United States, yet there is a minimal awareness of stroke as a major illness," says Dr. JoAnn Manson, co-investigator of the Nurses' Health Study.

This is a matter of deep concern for women because the stroke rate, which had been dropping, is believed to be on the rise. This is because the female population is getting older. In addition, due to advances in treatment, more women are surviving the heart attacks that once would have killed them, and are left with damaged hearts, which heightens stroke risk.

Mortality figures don't tell the whole story. Stroke is the most common crippler of women. Many people say they'd prefer to die of a heart attack than cancer (as if we're given a choice), but no one says that about stroke. Stroke is greatly feared, as well it should be. It can render your arms and legs useless, your speech unintelligible, your thoughts garbled. In an instant, stroke can transform a capable woman into a helpless invalid. If a person has a heart attack, maybe they can't run up the stairs as fast as they used to, but when they recover, they are usually able to resume most of their activities. This is not true of the person who has a stroke. It is estimated that only 10 percent of stroke victims recover all their abilities.

The real tragedy, though, is that stroke is thought of as inevitable; in fact, it is one of the most preventable causes not only of death but of disability and human suffering.

TWO TYPES OF STROKE

There are two broad categories of strokes. *Ischemic strokes* occur when too little blood flows to the brain. *Hemorrhagic strokes* occur when there is bleeding in the brain.

Ischemic Strokes

These strokes, caused by blood clots in the brain, are the most common type, making up about 80 percent of all strokes. They are also the most preventable. The following types of stroke fall within the broad category of ischemic strokes.

Cerebral Thrombosis

This type accounts for at least half of all strokes suffered. It is caused by a clot (also known as a *thrombus*) that builds up in the artery of the brain. Usually it is caused by the same factors that cause coronary heart disease.

Cerebral Embolism

This accounts for 30 percent of all strokes. Like cerebral thrombosis, it is also caused by a blockage; however, the clot does not build up in the artery itself but is swept into the brain from elsewhere in the body, such as the heart or the lungs.

Hemorrhagic Strokes

Hemorrhagic strokes, caused by bleeding, usually result when a weakened blood vessel in the brain bursts. Far less common than ischemic strokes, they usually are fatal and, if not, cause devastating brain damage. There are two types of hemorrhagic strokes:

Cerebral Hemorrhage

This type is the result of an *aneurysm*, a ruptured small blood vessel that has weakened, balloons out, and bursts. High blood pressure can cause such a stroke.

Subarachnoid Hemorrhage

This type is most often due to the bursting of an aneurysm on the surface of the brain. The result is an excruciating headache, often followed by coma, caused by pressure on the brain as the blood is trapped between the brain and the skull.

FACTORS THAT INCREASE YOUR RISK OF A STROKE

Growing Older

We associate stroke with old age, and this is generally true. After 55, the risk of stroke more than doubles with each passing decade. In fact, two-thirds of all strokes occur in people over the age of 65.

Women have an advantage in the case of stroke that is similar to their gender protection for heart disease. They tend to be six to ten years older than men when they suffer a stroke. This is not always an advantage, though. In fact, a stroke can be devastating to women in their seventies and eighties because they are more frail and less likely to recover.

Not only old people suffer strokes. An estimated 28 percent of stroke victims are under the age of 65. Glenda, a 43-year-old journalist, was seemingly in robust health when she slumped over at her mother's kitchen table, unconscious. The culprit was an aneurysm that caused a hemorrhagic stroke. Emergency surgery saved her life. The cause was a congenital malformation of some of the brain's blood vessels. "Apparently, I've had this since I was born, like a time bomb," she said.

Strokes in the young and middle-aged, while uncommon, are not extraordinary. Stroke does occur only in five to six out of a thousand people in their thirties. But this translates to up to 70,000 people being stricken every year. Hemorrhagic strokes are more common; although they constitute only 20 percent of strokes, they make up half of those strokes that occur in younger people.

When younger women are stricken by stroke, it's often due to such reasons as being born with abnormal blood vessels or defects, rare complications of childbirth, ulcerative colitis, Crohn's disease, rheumatoid arthritis, or AIDS. Such occurrences are not common, but they do happen.

Race

All women are at risk for stroke, no matter what their race or ethnic group, but African-American women are at the highest risk, even when they're young. In fact, at the age of 45 they have quadruple the risk. After that their risk gradually declines, and by the time they reach 85, it is slightly lower than that of white women. However, at all ages an African-American woman who suffers a stroke is twice as likely to die as her white counterpart.

It's believed the stroke risk for African-American women is so high because they are more likely to develop high blood pressure, the deadliest of risk factors. Stroke can also occur as a complication of sickle-cell anemia, an inherited blood disease to which African-Americans (and, less often, people of Mediterranean origin) are prone. Even teenagers with sickle-cell anemia can suffer strokes.

Family Medical History

Your risk of having a stroke increases if you have one or more close family members who have suffered a stroke. However, the role genetics plays in stroke is complicated and not completely understood.

In a study of twins published in the journal *Stroke* in 1992, siblings whose identical twins suffered a stroke were five times more likely to suffer one themselves than if they were fraternal twins. Since identical twins share the same genetic cellular makeup, this points to a strong genetic connection.

This twin study focused on men who suffered strokes as a result of atherosclerosis, the narrowing of the arteries that, when it occurs in the heart, results in heart disease, and when it occurs in the brain, causes stroke. Since the factors that contribute to atherosclerosis are similar in men and women, the results of this study should apply to women as well.

If stroke runs in your family, you need to find out what type it is. For instance, if your relatives suffered strokes due to aneurysms, you need to consult a neurologist to determine if you may have inherited this condition. If, on the other hand, your relatives suffered strokes due to abnormal blood cholesterol levels or high blood pressure, you should be monitored for these conditions.

If stroke is common in your family, you should begin screening while you're young and have tests done as often as your doctor deems necessary. If stroke is very prevalent in your family, consider consulting a neurologist who specializes in genetics. Invite your relatives along. You can find such a specialist by contacting the neurology department of a major medical center.

High Blood Pressure

High blood pressure is the most common—and important—stroke risk factor, experts concur. Statistics have shown that an estimated 50 to 75 percent of stroke victims have high blood pressure.

How does having high blood pressure increase your stroke risk? Your blood flows through your body in accordance with a pressurized system. Pressure that is too high damages the delicate vessels in the brain, causing atherosclerosis, which narrows the blood vessels of the brain and can result in blood clots, aneurysm, or a spontaneous rupture, causing a stroke.

When blood pressure is checked, two values are recorded. The higher one occurs when the heart contracts (systole); the lower occurs when the heart relaxes between beats (diastole). Blood pressure is written as systolic pressure followed by a slash followed by the diastolic pressure: for example, 120/80 mm (millimeters of mercury). This reading is read aloud as "one- twenty over eighty."

In a type of high blood pressure known as *isolated systolic hypertension*, the systolic pressure is 140 mm Hg (millimeters of mercury) or more, but the diastolic pressure is less than 90 mm Hg, that is, it is in the range of normal. Since blood pressure increases with age, this type is common in the elderly and was once thought to be harmless. However, recent studies have shown that this isn't true; elevated blood pressure, whether it is systolic, diastolic, or both, should be treated to lower stroke risk.

Beat Your Risk: *Although treating high blood pressure is extremely important, it doesn't eliminate stroke risk completely. So if you have high blood pressure—even if it's well controlled—you must stay on guard and recognize any warning signs.*

Smoking

Smoking is second only to high blood pressure in posing the greatest risk factor for all types of stroke. The Nurses' Health Study found that smoking can increase the risk of stroke in women up to four times. In fact, women who smoke have been found to be at even higher risk for stroke than male smokers. Smoking has also been found to be a risk factor for strokes that occur in younger women.

The more you smoke, the greater your risk. A woman who smokes 40 cigarettes a day is almost twice as likely to have a stroke as a 10-cigarette-a-day smoker, studies show.

Exactly how does tobacco smoke contribute to stroke? A stroke occurs when the brain is unable to receive enough blood. Inhaling cigarette smoke produces a number of effects that can impact the flow of blood to the brain. Carbon monoxide, when it gets into the blood, reduces the amount of oxygen that reaches the brain. Cigarette smoke also contributes to the narrowing of the vessels that bring blood to the brain, just as it damages the heart's coronary arteries. Furthermore, the nicotine in cigarettes contains substances that make the blood more likely to clot, which can cause a stroke.

As if this wasn't bad enough, smoking contributes to the risk of hemorrhagic stroke, caused by blood leaking into the brain. Although it's not known how smoking causes this, it may be that inhaling nicotine causes blood pressure to suddenly spike, which can burst a blood vessel.

Smoking and Taking Oral Contraceptives

When first developed, oral contraceptives were found to increase stroke risk. Over the years the amount of hormones they contain have lessened, and so has the risk. However, cigarette smoke and oral con-traceptives independently contain clotting factors that when com-bined, dramatically increase the risk of a stroke.

Heart Disease and Other Heart Problems

Any irregularity in the flow of blood to the brain can cause it to clot, resulting in a stroke. Sometimes this occurs because of heart disease or another type of heart problem. The following are the car-diac-related causes of stroke.

Bear in mind that heart disease, irregular heartbeats, and cardiac valve problems are the more common types of cardiac causes of stroke. Strokes caused by congenital heart defects and cardiac tu-mors are much more rare, but they do occur.

Heart Disease

Emily, whose story was related at the beginning of this chapter, suffered her stroke following a heart attack. "I had no idea that a heart attack could lead to this," she said. But it can, and it all too often does.

Heart disease can set the stage for a stroke in two ways. First, heart disease results in the narrowing of the coronary arteries, but if this process is occurring in your heart's arteries, it's also happening in your brain. The flow of blood to the brain can be impeded, and eventually blocked. The result is a stroke. Second, this atheroscle-rotic process also causes blood clots. If a blood clot originates in the heart and travels to the brain, that also can result in a stroke.

Irregular Heartbeats (Atrial Fibrillation)

Your heartbeat is governed by the electrical system of your heart. A heart attack, for instance, can damage this system, and an irregular heartbeat can result. Atrial fibrillation is a type of heartbeat irregularity that steeply raises the risk of stroke. In fact, about 15 percent of strokes are believed to result from this problem.

In atrial fibrillation, the upper chambers of the heart beat too rapidly. This fluttery quivering isn't forceful enough to send all the blood through to the heart's lower chambers, as it should. As a result, the blood can pool, forming a clot that travels to the brain and causes a stroke.

Atrial fibrillation commonly occurs in women over the age of 70 and increases their stroke risk fivefold. Strokes in elderly women with this condition also cause more permanent disability.

The use of such anticoagulants as aspirin and Coumadin, a powerful blood thinner, reduce the risk of this type of stroke. But such treatment is used too little, some experts estimate. Treatment could prevent 50 to 80 percent of the strokes caused by this ailment.

Heart Valve Problems

The proper flow of blood through your heart depends on your four cardiac valves. These can stiffen with age, causing them to operate improperly. If the flow of blood is disrupted, a clot can form. If it travels to the brain, the result is a stroke. Women who had rheumatic fever as children can develop cardiac valve problems later in life. So can women with artificial heart valves. They usually take Coumadin to prevent this.

Congenital Heart Defects

The heart begins to form a single tubelike structure during conception. For unknown reasons, the heart can fail to form properly, and the result is a congenital heart defect. One type, called a *septal defect*, results in a hole in the heart's chamber. If it is not severe, it can remain undetected. If it does, the blood flows improperly through the body and bypasses the lungs, which normally filter out tiny clots. If a clot remains, it can travel to the brain, resulting in a stroke. Such defects can be surgically repaired, eliminating the risk of stroke.

Cardiac Tumors

Primary tumors in the heart are rare, and when they do occur, are usually benign. However, even if it is harmless, a tiny bit can break off from the tumor, travel in the bloodstream to the brain, and result in a stroke.

Beat Your Risk: *Sometimes a stroke is the first clue to an undiagnosed heart problem. If you have a stroke, ask to be examined for heart disease. If it's not found and treated, you could suffer a heart attack. A subsequent heart attack is the most common cause of death in women who have suffered a stroke.*

Diabetes

Diabetes, whether Type I or Type II, sharply increases the risk of stroke, in two ways. First, as noted in chapter 11, this disorder sets the stage for heart disease, a major stroke risk factor. Just as diabetes erases your so-called gender protection from heart disease, it does so for stroke. Women between the ages of 40 and 60 are unlikely to suffer a stroke— unless they are diabetic. For diabetic women, the rate of stroke increases to that of men.

Second, the higher blood-glucose levels found in diabetics can weaken the brain's delicate blood vessels, causing a stroke. Diabetic women are also more likely to develop high blood pressure, which raises stroke risk even higher.

Beat Your Risk: *If you are diabetic, it is even more important that you have your blood pressure checked frequently and, if you develop high blood pressure, control it firmly. Blood-pressure levels that might be deemed within normal limits in nondiabetics are not considered acceptable in diabetics because they are more prone to suffer damage from it.*

Oral Contraceptives

After birth-control pills came on the market 25 years ago, eventually it became known that the high doses of estrogen they contained were linked to a variety of undesirable effects, particularly stroke. Since then birth-control pills have been reformulated and the amount of estrogen reduced. Although this hasn't eradicated all of the health concerns, it has reduced them.

However, there may be some exceptions. One is for women who smoke and take the Pill. A study published in 1996 in the *New England Journal of Medicine* looked at 295 women between the ages of 15 and 44 who had suffered a stroke between 1991 and 1994. This study was designed to evaluate the risk of stroke in smokers using the new lower-dose estrogen birth-control pills. The study didn't find any increased risk for nonsmokers; however, the risk was increased for women who smoked.

Beat Your Risk: *Both cigarette smoke and oral contraceptives contain their own clotting mechanisms that, when combined, can raise a female smoker's risk of stroke 22 times, according to the American Heart Association. The risk may be lower for women who take low-estrogen pills, but the extent is not known.*

OTHER FACTORS

What about Cholesterol?

Cholesterol is linked with heart attacks. Is there a connection with stroke, too? Yes, but the link is fuzzier.

Although people with high blood cholesterol do run a two- to threefold increased risk of ischemic stroke, people with the lowest blood cholesterol level have a higher rate of hemorrhagic stroke, according to the American Heart Association. The results of clinical trials using cholesterol-lowering drugs have also been mixed, with some drugs showing a reduction in stroke risk and others a troubling increase.

Pregnancy

Pregnancy is not usually thought of as a risk factor for stroke, but such complications can occur. During pregnancy, changes occur in the chemistry of the blood that increase its clotting ability. Therefore, pregnant women are at increased risk for stroke from blood clots and remain so during the first several weeks after giving birth.

Bear in mind that pregnant women do not have a high stroke rate. However, women who have experienced six or more strokes are at increased risk. This is apparently not due to the pregnancies themselves, but because these women have a tendency to develop insulin resistance (a metabolic condition related to diabetes), and diabetes is a major contributor to stroke in women.

Symptoms of stroke during pregnancy include headache, nausea, vomiting, seizures, and loss of consciousness. If you experience such symptoms, contact your doctor.

Can a Migraine Cause a Stroke?

"My headaches are so unbearable I often feel I am going to have a stroke. My friends pooh-pooh this idea, but are they wrong?" wonders Christie, a 32-year-old publicist.

Because migraines can temporarily cause symptoms that are similar to stroke, including intense head pain, slurred speech, and numbness, it's not surprising that women who get severe migraines may fear they're going to have a stroke. And in fact, some studies have found that women who get migraines are four times more likely to suffer from a stroke, though this result has not been found consistently. Statistically, this means that as many as 10,000 Americans may suffer from a stroke-related migraine annually. Bear in mind, though, that the number of Americans who suffer from migraine numbers in the millions.

Exactly how migraines cause stroke is not known, but there are some possible explanations. In a migraine, the blood vessels of the brain narrow or widen. When they narrow, the blood flow is decreased. If this occurs, a clot may form. Another theory is that as the blood vessels in the brain contract, they secrete a chemical that is a clotting substance. Either factor could cause a stroke.

Studies find that increased stroke risk is not evenly distributed among all migraine sufferers. The types of migraine fall into two major groups: migraine without aura, known as *common migraine*, and migraine with aura, known as *classic migraine*. An aura is a group of symptoms that occur 20 to 60 minutes prior to the onset of the intense head pain that characterizes migraine.

Four out of five people with migraine experience migraine without aura; typically, their migraine is intense pain, often on one side of the head, although sometimes both. This can be accompanied by nausea and vomiting.

However, the remaining one-fifth experience aura with their migraine. Most auras involve visual problems, such as blurriness or partial blindness. Other manifestations are confusion or speech problems, such as difficulty finding the right word. Less commonly, migraine sufferers experience auras that include motor problems, such as partial paralysis or a feeling of weakness or heaviness in the limbs on one side of the body. This group is believed to be at higher risk for stroke.

Women who get migraines are also at additional risk if they have other risk factors for stroke, such as high blood pressure or heart disease. Most important among them, several studies have consistently found, are migraine sufferers who smoke and take birth-control pills. This has been found to be true especially for women under the age of 35. If you get migraines, contact your doctor if you experience any of these warning signs:

- If you experience neurological symptoms that are unusual for you
- If your aura lasts longer than usual, or if you suddenly begin to experience paralysis along with them
- If you're over 40 years old, and you're experiencing what appears to be a migraine and/or aura symptoms for the first time. In this case, don't assume you're having a migraine; call your doctor.

Remember, stroke is a rare complication of migraine. But if you get migraines, it makes sense to reduce any stroke risk factors you may have.

Osteoporosis and Stroke: A Connection?

Osteoporosis increases the risk of stroke, studies have found. The worse the osteoporosis, the more likely the stroke. The connection isn't precisely known, but it may be because women who have osteoporosis also have low levels of estrogen in their blood after menopause, and this may increase the risk of stroke.

Hormone Replacement Therapy

Generally, women suffer both heart attacks and strokes later in life than do men, a difference generally termed gender protection. Since this gender difference in heart disease is ascribed to estrogen, and there is considerable evidence that replacing this hormone after menopause cuts heart disease rates, it makes sense to look at this issue for stroke as well.

Fewer studies on stroke have been done, and the results are conflicting. Some studies do find a beneficial effect, although not as dramatic a reduction as in heart disease. In any case, more research needs to be completed before a definite conclusion can be drawn. For more information, see chapter 18.

Stroke as a Surgical Complication

When her 64-year-old mother-in-law, Marie, went into the hospital for bypass surgery, Sally wasn't too worried. "People have coronary bypass surgery all the time. My father had it last year, and it went great. So I'm sure it will go fine," she said. Sally was heartbroken when Marie suffered a stroke during the second day of her recuperation.

Certain cardiac procedures have become so commonplace that we tend to take them for granted. But these treatments, which involve the heart and its blood vessels, do carry the risk of a stroke. This includes any open-heart surgery, as well as less invasive procedures to widen narrowed blood vessels such as angioplasty and atherectomy. Even cardiac catheterization, a commonly performed diagnostic procedure, carries with it a slight stroke risk.

Although such strokes occur rarely, women are at slightly more risk for them, possibly because we have smaller arteries, and because heart disease in women may be more advanced when it is diagnosed and is more likely to be treated on an emergency basis.

These strokes are often unavoidable. But put the odds in your favor. If you are told you need one of these cardiac procedures, proceed cautiously. Get a second opinion (or even a third) if you have any doubt. Select the doctor and the hospital where it is to be performed carefully. Generally, the institutions that do the largest number of cardiac procedures have the best survival rates and the lowest rates of serious complications such as stroke.

HOW TO REDUCE YOUR RISK OF A STROKE

Control Your High Blood Pressure

If there is stroke in your family medical history, or you have other risk factors that raise the odds, have your blood pressure checked frequently. Should you develop high blood pressure, follow your doctor's recommendations to control it. Sometimes high blood pressure can be controlled with diet and exercise; sometimes medication is also needed. Whatever the case, controlling blood pressure is important, because it can decrease your stroke risk by 40 percent or more.

Quit Smoking

When you quit smoking, your added risk of stroke diminishes and eventually will decrease to that of a woman who never smoked.

This was demonstrated in a study published in 1993 in the *Journal of the American Medical Association*, which looked at the stroke risk of 117,006 women. The research found that the extra risk of former smokers for stroke largely disappeared two to four years after quitting, and it didn't matter how long the women had smoked or how heavily.

Eat Lots of Fruits and Vegetables

Scientists are identifying several factors that can influence whether you suffer a stroke. Consuming ample amounts of vegetables appears to lower stroke risk in women, according to research presented by Dr. JoAnn Manson, co-investigator of the Nurses' Health Study. At a 1993 American Heart Association meeting, she and her colleagues reviewed the medical history and food habits of the study's participants. Those who ate the most vegetables, particularly carrots and spinach, had the lowest risk of stroke.

Exactly how fruits and vegetables are protective isn't known. One theory relates to homocysteine, the amino acid referred to earlier. High levels of that amino acid in the blood have been linked to an increased risk of both heart attack and stroke in elderly and middle-aged men and possibly in women as well. Folic acid, contained in the B vitamins, helps lower homocysteine levels. Potassium may help lower risk as well. These substances are found in fruits and vegetables, so take a stroll down the produce aisle.

Get Moving!

Exercise reduces the risk of many conditions that set the stage for stroke, including heart disease, diabetes, and high blood pressure. A study published in 1996 in the *American Journal of Epidemiology* noted that this positive benefit was found for stroke risk even when factoring out these other diseases. This study is similar to others that show exercise is beneficial, including the Nurses' Health Study, which showed that the most active women cut their stroke risk by 42 percent.

STROKE: A "BRAIN ATTACK"

Not long ago, a person suffering a stroke was not seen as in need of urgent medical care. Indeed, it was believed that the stroke had to "run its course" and nothing could be done to mitigate the resulting brain damage. Difficult as it is to believe nowadays, that was once the view of heart attacks as well: that a person's condition could be stabilized, but there was nothing to do to halt the damage.

This viewpoint about stroke is changing as treatments are developed that will both stop a stroke and halt the damage that results. Because of this progress, stroke is now thought of as a "brain attack," warranting immediate attention.

Even doctors lack stroke awareness. Every year 35,000 people suffer strokes while they are hospitalized. These patients would be ideal candidates for early intervention, but stroke symptoms in these patients often go unrecognized even by hospital personnel, a study published in 1993 in the journal *Stroke* found.

Prompt diagnosis and treatment of stroke is needed to:

• Reduce the risk of death. Stroke is the third leading cause of death, but if you get to a hospital early enough, you are less likely to die from the stroke itself or from life-threatening complications such as pneumonia.

• Benefit from the latest stroke treatments, which must be given within hours. These include drugs known as clot busters that can halt the damage from stroke

• Reduce the risk of a second stroke, which can follow on the heels of the first and be the one that causes death or major damage

• Reduce the risk of life-threatening complications, such as pneumonia

Prompt diagnosis is also needed because sometimes what seems to be a stroke isn't one at all. Low blood sugar in diabetics, a brain tumor, or even a treatable brain infection can cause the same symptoms as stroke. "As scary as the thought of a stroke is, what is even scarier is not to treat a problem that may have been treatable," notes Dr. Brass.

Beat Your Risk: *If you believe you may be suffering a stroke and seek medical help, have the emergency room staff contact your regular doctor. A doctor who is familiar with you may be able to recognize subtle abnormalities, such as a weakness in your hand, that might otherwise be overlooked. If you have suffered a stroke in the past, make sure that your neurologist is notified.*

THE WARNING SIGNS OF STROKE

Of all the risk factors for stroke, perhaps the greatest is ignorance. A survey commissioned by the American Heart Association showed that only 43 percent of the respondents could name even one of the several warning signs of stroke and only 29 percent would get immediate help for certain stroke symptoms. But knowing these warning signs could save your life.

Stroke warning signs are:

- Sudden weakness or numbness of the face, arm, or leg on one side of the body
- Sudden difficulty speaking or understanding others
- Dimness or impaired vision, particularly in only one eye or half of both eyes
- Confusion, which comes on suddenly
- Sudden unexplained dizziness
- Sudden onset of unsteadiness or lack of coordination, difficulty walking, or falling
- Sudden excruciating headache
- Recent change in personality or mental abilities, including memory loss

---

Beat Your Risk: You should be aware that while sometimes a stroke comes on with little or no warning, many times they progress over several hours; first the victim may become dizzy, for example, then notice her vision dimming, and finally begin experiencing paralysis. Don't wait; summon help immediately.

THE "BRAIN ATTACK" WARNING SIGNAL: TRANSIENT ISCHEMIC ATTACKS

A *transient ischemic attack* (TIA), also known as a mini-stroke, is a serious warning sign of an impending stroke and must not be ignored. It can be compared to angina, the classic chest pain that warns of a looming heart attack.

The symptoms of a TIA are the same as a stroke, but its duration can be fleeting, lasting from several minutes to a half hour, and easy to brush aside. But anyone who experiences symptoms that may be a TIA should get immediate medical help. Treatments are available to reduce the risk of a major stroke, so such a warning sign should be heeded. If you are suffering stroke symptoms or TIAs, experts recommend that you contact the neurological department at a large medical center instead of your small community hospital. The field has grown so rapidly that the problem is not only that patients and the general public are poorly educated but the general physician as well. Studies show you can get quicker treatment by calling 911 instead of your family physician.

Beat Your Risk: *Remember that a TIA can have the same warning signs as a stroke yet be fleeting. If this happens to you, resist the urge to brush it aside. Get help.*

THE BOTTOM LINE

Strokes pose a threat to women, killing twice the number that breast cancer does, yet it remains a nearly invisible problem. Although mostly older women, in their seventies and eighties, suffer strokes, younger women can as well. Adopting healthy eating and exercise regimens can help reduce the risk of a stroke. Also, learning the warning signs of stroke and getting immediate help is extremely important in conquering the odds of this leading killer and crippler of women.

Rate Your Risk: Stroke

Put a check mark after each answer. Answer all questions. Then consult the scoring key to compute your score.

	Score	
	(+ column)	(– column)

Family History

1. Do you have a close relative who has _____ _____
   suffered a stroke?

   Yes_____ +1   No _____ 0

Personal History/Habits

2. What is your age? _____ _____

   Under 55   _____+1

   Between 55 and 65   _____+2

   Over 65   _____+3

3. Is the systolic reading (the upper _____ _____
   number) of your blood pressure
   consistently above 160?

   Yes_____ +4   No _____ 0

4. Do you smoke? _____ _____

   Yes_____ +3   No _____ 0

5. Do you smoke and take oral _____ _____
   contraceptives?

   Yes_____ +5   No _____ 0

6. Have you ever had any of the _____ _____
   following: heart attack, chest pain
   caused by heart disease, narrowed
   coronary blood vessels, narrowed
   arteries in the legs, or congestive
   heart failure?

   Yes_____ +3   No _____ 0

7. Do you have a history of atrial
   fibrillation (a specific type of rapid,
   irregular heartbeat)?
   Yes_____ +3   No _____ 0
8. Do you have diabetes?
   Yes_____ +2   No _____ 0
9. Are you generally physically inactive?
   Yes_____ +1   No _____ 0
      Subtotal
      Risk Factor   +5
      (add in only if you answered
      yes to all or either #5, 6, or 7)
      Final Score

How to Score

1. Fill in the numbers in the columns at the far right.
2. Add the +5 if you answered yes to a particular risk factor.
3. Subtotal your score.
4. Compute your final score.
5. Compare your score to the Risk Factor Scoring Chart.

Stroke Risk Factor Scoring Chart

   Below 5   Lowest risk
   6 to 10   Low to moderate
   11 to 15   Moderate to high
   Above 16   Highest risk

Part Three

FOUR STEPS TO
REDUCING
YOUR RISKS

CHAPTER 15

STEP 1: QUIT SMOKING

WHEN LINDA WAS 12, her mother was diagnosed with heart disease. "She threw her cartons of cigarettes in the trash, and I fished them out and started smoking," Linda recalls. Her mother never did quit, and she died of a heart attack at the age of 42. Linda, continuing to smoke, built a three-pack-a-day habit. At just 28 she suffered a heart attack.

Her denim cap set at a jaunty angle, Pat was enjoying what appeared to be a simple lawn party. But this party was being held on the lawn of a hospital and was in honor of "cancer survivor" day. And a survivor is precisely what Pat, who has lung cancer, is hoping to be.

Rose was a busy woman, always involved with one charity or the other. She had no health problems she knew of, yet a massive stroke killed her suddenly at the age of 66.

Linda, Pat, and Rose had only one habit in common—smoking.

Smoking is strongly linked to almost all of the deadly killer diseases outlined in this book. No other risk factor that we can control can make that claim, or even come close.

Beat Your Risk: *If you are a smoker, and you make no other lifestyle change outlined in this book than to quit smoking, you will have taken the most important step in saving your life.*

HOW MANY WOMEN SMOKE?

Millions of American women smoke, and fewer have managed to kick the habit than have men. That women smoke so much can be largely attributed to the success of advertising. During the early 1900s, few women smoked. The habit was limited to the very rich or those women who were considered indecent. In the 1920s, tobacco companies refused to promote cigarettes directly to women for fear of a prohibitionist backlash. But during the Roaring Twenties, smoking gained ground among female college students and women who considered themselves trendsetters.

Men began smoking heavily during World War I, but not until World War II did large numbers of women take up the habit. At first they smoked less and did not inhale as deeply. As time passed, they began smoking more like men, at a younger age and more heavily. And their health risks mounted.

In 1964, when the surgeon general issued a landmark warning on the link between smoking and cancer, 50 percent of American men and 32 percent of women smoked. Over the years that rate has fallen, and now stands at a stable 25 percent for both men and women, despite the government's goal to persuade more to quit. The latest tally, announced by the federal Centers for Disease Control in 1998, found that, among women, the highest percentages of smokers are among American Indians and Alaska Natives (35.4 percent) and the lowest are among Asians and Pacific Islanders (4.3 percent). Rates were 24.1 percent, 23.5 percent, and 14.9 percent among whites, blacks, and Latinas, respectively. In another report, released in 1996, the government noted that teenage smoking has climbed to 34.8 from 27.5 percent five years ago. So there is a new population of smokers to replace the millions who die annually from smoking-related disease.

Beat Your Risk: *If you smoke, consider the role model you are setting for your daughter and quit. Studies find the parent whose smoking behavior is most likely to influence whether a girl will smoke is her mother.*

SMOKING IS A FEMINIST ISSUE

"When Tempted, Reach for a Lucky Instead," says one vintage newspaper ad, urging women to avoid a double chin by reaching for a cigarette. "She Wouldn't Smoke a Boring Cigarette," said another ad, years later. Then there's that unfortunately successful modern-day smoking campaign for Virginia Slims that intones, "You've Come a Long Way, Baby." The cigarette maker recently changed that motto to read, "It's a Woman Thing." Yeah, so is lung cancer now, unfortunately.

Even today many women fail to realize just how hazardous smoking is to their health. And don't expect the tobacco companies to tell them. They have worked long, hard, and successfully to portray just the opposite image.

"Women have been told for over fifty years that smoking is glamorous and sophisticated," said then Surgeon General Antonia Novello in 1991. The tobacco industry spent $3.3 billion to promote their product while far outspending the government's $3.5 million antismoking efforts, she noted.

If smoking is so dangerous to a woman's health, you might wonder why you don't read more about it in women's magazines. An answer to that question comes from Dr. Kenneth Warner, professor of health management and policy at the University of Michigan School of Public Health, who has written that magazines that accept cigarette advertising are more likely to practice self-censorship and not print articles about its dangers. He found this is particularly true of women's magazines.

Furthermore, tobacco companies often sponsor sporting events, cultural activities, and pursuits undertaken by women and minority groups. The most well-known of these is the Virginia Slims tennis tournament, and there have been others, such as national tours of the Joffrey Ballet and the More Fashion Awards, named after the cigarette brand.

Tobacco companies contribute generously to women's organizations and have successfully linked smoking with women's emancipation and equality with men, just as they've tried to link smoker's "rights" to our national Bill of Rights.

Tobacco companies also have targeted women by using special packaging for feminine appeal, introducing "designer" cigarettes and half-size packs perfect for slipping into a teenage girl's purse, and offering discounted women's products with the purchase of a particular brand of cigarettes. This is nothing new, as satirist Gary Trudeau notes in a Doonesbury comic strip. In the strip it's recounted that in 1934, when it was found that Lucky Strikes weren't selling well, marketers convened to find out why. It was learned that the women didn't like the color of the packaging, so the tobacco company undertook a massive fashion campaign to make green the fashion that season. Sad to say, it worked.

The tobacco industry's most brilliant strategy—which began over a half century ago and continues to this day—is the exploitation of women's fears about gaining weight. Back then cigarettes were advertised blatantly with the slogan "Reach for a Lucky Instead of a Sweet." Nowadays, the incorporation of the word "slims" into so many cigarette brands isn't done just to describe the shape of the cigarette—there's a more subtle message. There is some truth that smoking helps women weigh less. On the average, smokers weigh less than nonsmokers, and women frequently cite their fear of gaining weight as the reason they don't quit smoking. But this is a steep price to pay for dying prematurely!

Beat Your Risk: *Smoking does keep weight down, which is a major reason many women smoke, but it has other less desirable effects. Odor clinging to your clothes, nicotine-stained teeth, facial wrinkles, and crow's feet, for instance. Use this mental image as ammunition to help you quit!*

HOW SMOKING KILLS WOMEN

The specific information on how smoking affects the diseases in this book is discussed in those chapters, but here's a brief recap.

Breast Cancer

The evidence on whether smoking cigarettes contributes to breast cancer is contradictory, but research does show that if you smoke and you develop breast cancer, you're more likely to die.

Cervical Cancer

When you smoke, you inhale toxins that enter your bloodstream and travel to your cervix. It's believed that these poisons may mix with harmless bacteria in the cervix that then become carcinogenic and/or the toxins inhibit the normal cancer-fighting immune response of the cells in the cervix.

Colon Cancer

Smoking is a clearly established risk factor in male smokers and is thought to be one in women as well. Although it's not known exactly how smoking raises the risk of colon cancer, the rate of this disease in women is rising and is clearly correlated with the rate in which women took up smoking in this country.

Lung Cancer

It's estimated that a whopping 80 percent of all lung cancer cases are directly attributable to smoking. Smoking envelopes the lungs in scores of carcinogens and toxic gases, and the end result is lung cancer, which is among the most common—and deadliest—types of cancer in women. Smoking is also directly responsible for the sharp increase in such lung diseases as emphysema.

Diabetes

Women smokers have higher rates of diabetes. Although it's not known exactly why, smoking raises both blood glucose levels and insulin resistance, two markers for this disease. This correlation is also "dose dependent," which means the heavier the smoker, the higher the risk.

Heart Disease

Women who smoke have a far greater risk of heart disease and heart attack; in fact, smoking erases the so-called gender protection women have against these killers in their younger years. Cigarette smoke damages the heart's coronary arteries, which bring blood to the heart, and causes clotting, which can result in a heart attack. Female smokers who take oral contraceptives have a greatly increased risk of heart attack.

Osteoporosis

Women who smoke are much more likely to develop osteoporosis; it's believed that the poisons in cigarette smoke interfere with the metabolic processes needed to create strong bones.

Stroke

Female smokers are estimated to have a tripled risk of stroke. Cigarette smoke damages the delicate blood vessels in the brain, diminishes the amount of needed oxygen in the blood, and causes clotting, which leads to stroke. As with heart disease, female smokers who take oral contraceptives have a far greater risk of stroke.

HOW TO QUIT SMOKING

So there are plenty of reasons to quit smoking, but the question remains: how do you do it?

According to a study done by the Centers for Disease Control, 73 percent of female smokers want to quit but don't because they are addicted. There's also some evidence that women may find it more difficult to quit, says Cynthia S. Pomerleau, Ph.D., director of the University of Michigan's nicotine research laboratory. "It always raises a certain amount of controversy when it's said, but large studies show that the quit rate in women is consistently lower than that in men," she said.

Smoking is exceptionally difficult to overcome because it has not only a physiological but a psychological aspect as well. Smoking becomes an ingrained habit in response with behavioral cues, for example, having a cigarette with that first cup of coffee at breakfast or while watching television at night. "Nicotine has a strong effect in terms of addiction, but the behavioral component gives it a double whammy," notes Dr. Pomerleau. Remember Linda, the woman whose story was recounted at the beginning of this chapter? Her memories of her mother are intertwined with smoking.

"After my mother was diagnosed with heart disease, she was in denial, and she didn't stop smoking. I started smoking too, and I remember we would sit together at the table, drink coffee, smoking cigarettes, and talk together," she recalls.

Also, that dose of nicotine simply makes us feel good. The effects of nicotine are fast and predictable. "Although the effects on mood and performance are small, they're very reliable, so you can get them virtually on demand," Dr. Pomerleau notes.

Beat Your Risk: Some women who find it impossible to quit smoking are clinically depressed or suffer from anxiety disorder, and smoking helps keep these symptoms at bay. If you think you may be in this group, consider getting additional help, such as psychological counseling and/or medication, before you try to quit smoking.

TEN TIPS TO QUIT SMOKING

It's important to have a plan in place before you try to quit. This helps because you can anticipate the obstacles that may arise and prepare a strategy ahead of time to overcome them.

Remember, studies find that men and women smoke for different reasons. While both genders smoke to deal with stress, for example, women use cigarettes to help control their weight. If you understand the problems that may arise while you're quitting, you can come up with potential solutions.

1. Find a Buddy

Finding a friend who sincerely wants to quit smoking can be valuable, just as dieting with a friend can be. But even if you don't have such a friend, there are other options; you can find other people who want to quit smoking at a smoking-cessation program or check the Internet for support groups in cyberspace.

2. Be Realistic about Your Weight

Most women smoke to control their weight. About 20 percent of women don't gain weight if they try to quit, but the majority gain between 5 and 15 pounds. A majority—the supergainers, Dr. Pomerleau calls them—may put on 25 pounds, but this is very unusual. When she did a survey, most of the women said they were not willing to put on more than 5 pounds.

It's important to anticipate a possible gain in weight and determine ahead of time how to deal with it. Sometimes the weight gain happens because, since nicotine raises metabolism, smoking may have kept your weight unnaturally low. In addition, increased appetite can be part of the smoking-withdrawal process. If you understand all this ahead of time, you can anticipate that you may gain a little weight, but resolve that it won't upset you so much that you'll abandon your quitting plan. Instead you can see it as a temporary problem and plan to take the weight off later.

Dr. Pomerleau suggests that women wait for three months and see what their weight is. Then if they need to, they can take steps to lose it. Although it seems logical to add a weight-control program to stopping smoking, this apparently doesn't work, possibly because the stress of both dieting and quitting smoking is unbearable.

Another reason to put off worrying about weight for a few months is that you'll be able to exercise more easily later and can add that to a weight-control plan. "It's hard to get anybody to exercise. Smokers are not the easiest people to motivate because the smoking has compromised lung function. After you stop smoking, you can exercise better," Dr. Pomerleau said.

Reevaluate your ideas about weight. Do you have an unrealistic idea about what you should weigh? If you do, and you've been depending on cigarettes to keep your weight at an unnatural level, you may need to rethink your views on weight before you can deal with the prospect of gaining any—even temporarily.

3. Create "Stress-Busters"

Many women smoke as a way to manage stress. Practicing a stress-management technique, such as yoga or meditation, can be very helpful. A number of women find they need "to do something with their hands" to take the place of cigarettes. Knitting, rug hooking, and needlepoint are alternatives; just be certain you find these activities enjoyable, not stress-producing.

4. Consider Nicotine Replacement

Since smoking is addicting, it's not surprising that about 80 percent of those who quit experience some withdrawal symptoms, and there is some evidence that women experience them even more severely than men do. These symptoms can be intense for 2 or 3 days, but within 10 to 14 days after quitting, most usually subside. The most common withdrawal symptoms are:

- Depression
- Insomnia
- Irritability
- Frustration and/or anger

- Anxiety
- Difficulty concentrating
- Restlessness
- Appetite increase and weight gain

Whatever the reason, it can make quitting seem impossible. Although it's tempting to think that smokers can quit using sheer willpower, you may not be able to. In fact, some research suggests that women may need stronger nicotine replacement than men do.

In the past few years, a number of nicotine substitutes have been developed. Nicotine gum, which is available over the counter, is the drug in gum form. It releases small amounts of nicotine, which are absorbed by the body, cutting down on withdrawal symptoms. A nicotine patch is applied to your skin, and the drug enters your body gradually. The nicotine nasal spray delivers nicotine through the nose; the nicotine inhaler, into the mouth. Do they work? Generally, yes, particularly in people who are strongly addicted, such as those who crave a cigarette as soon as they awaken. With these aids, the amount of nicotine stays level in the body, so there are less severe cravings.

Another alternative is a prescription drug known as Zyban—a sustained-released tablet form of bupropion hydrochloride, which is marketed in another form as an antidepressant. The drug boosts the levels of two types of brain chemicals in the body, dopamine and norepinephrine, just as nicotine does. A study published in 1997 in the *New England Journal of Medicine* found that this pill worked as well as the nicotine substitutes.

These products don't remove all the difficulty from quitting, but they can ease it. Studies also find that the people who have the most success with these nicotine substitutes are those who use them in conjunction with counseling or a smoking-cessation program.

It's important to remember never to smoke when using a nicotine substitute because you could suffer a heart attack. In addition, if you've had a heart attack, nicotine in any form can be dangerous, so check with your doctor. Products containing nicotine are not advised for pregnant women because of its potential harm to the fetus.

Beat Your Risk: *Studies indicate that, because women may be more heavily addicted than men, they sometimes require more nicotine substitution. Since nicotine replacement systems allow for adjusting the dosage of the drug, you can do this. But don't take more than the recommended levels without first discussing it with your doctor.*

---

5. Pick the Right Time to Quit

It probably comes as no surprise to you that your hormones play a role in how you feel. Although studies find women don't smoke any more or less during the month, when they try to quit right before their period, or during it, many report worsened withdrawal symptoms. In addition, some women also crave cigarettes right before they get their period, so this is obviously not the best time during the month to quit. A better time to quit might be a few days after your period.

6. Prepare for Your "Quit Day"

You may have lots of friends who brag that they quit cold turkey. If you can do this, great. But don't be disheartened if you cannot—most research shows that this is very difficult to do. In a Canadian study published in 1994 in the journal *Women and Health*, 50 percent of the women in the research project had successfully stayed off cigarettes for over a year. This study found that a technique known as nicotine fading, in which the participants gradually switched over to cigarette brands progressively lower in tar and nicotine, was useful. In their book *How Women Can Finally Stop Smoking*, authors Robert C. Klesges, Ph.D., and Margaret DeBon, M.S., discuss choosing a specific day to quit. Although this sounds like quitting cold turkey, it actually isn't; the authors outline specific preparation to take before that day, including gradually decreasing the number of cigarettes you're smoking by 50 percent.

7. Eat Healthy Foods

Smokers often have bad nutritional habits; they tend to skip more meals, drink more coffee, and eat more sweets or junk foods than nonsmokers. Pay attention to nutrition. While dieting can be difficult during this time, concentrating on fruits, vegetables, and high-fiber foods that are filling can be useful. The Canadian study found that by eating several small meals throughout the day, the women were able to keep their blood sugar stable and their mood more calm and to resist cravings for sugar-laden candy and chocolate.

8. Cut Your Caffeine Intake in Half

Some smoking-cessation programs advise cutting out caffeine, particularly coffee, completely, reasoning that since so many people smoke and drink coffee at the same time, this helps break the habit. But caffeine, like nicotine, is also a stimulant with addictive qualities, and quitting can bring on withdrawal symptoms, including severe headache, that can also be unbearable. Klesges and DeBon note in their book that smoking reduces the stimulant qualities of caffeine by about half. So if your caffeine intake stays the same, you end up overdosing on it and experiencing the same type of edginess and shakiness that quitting smoking brings. Their solution: cut your caffeine intake in half.

9. Prepare for a Relapse

You are most vulnerable to relapse—and starting to smoke again—during the first few weeks after quitting. During this time there are four situations in which you are most vulnerable, according to Klesges and DeBon. They are:

- When you are emotionally upset
- When you are happy, particularly when you are particularly enjoying yourself in a social situation like a reunion or a holiday party

- During evening activities, especially when alcohol is available to cloud your resolve
- When you're bored

If you anticipate these situations and prepare ahead of time, you're less likely to relapse. For instance, if you're in a situation where alcohol is served, space out your drinks, alternate between alcoholic and nonalcoholic drinks, or limit yourself to a certain number of drinks.

Even if you relapse, this doesn't mean you're a permanent failure. According to the Canadian study, even if a woman relapsed and smoked an entire cigarette during the first week, this didn't necessarily doom her efforts. The authors speculated that slips are a normal part of learning to quit, and they demonstrate to the smoker how easy it would be to start smoking again. And remember that most people who successfully quit have failed at least once, maybe more!

10. Reward Yourself

Many people like to employ a "cigarette fund" to provide them with motivation. There are variations of this, but usually the money that would have been spent on cigarettes is set aside in a special jar. You can earmark that money for a trip, a special purchase, or another treat you wouldn't ordinarily buy for yourself.

FORMAL SMOKING-CESSATION PROGRAMS

If quitting on your own doesn't work, don't consider yourself a failure. Many people need the help of a formal program to carry through with their quitting plans. The American Heart Association, the American Lung Association, the American Cancer Society, and the Seventh Day Adventists all offer smoking-cessation programs. Bear in mind, though, that some programs are based on research that focused on men. So if you choose such a program, make sure it fulfills your needs. Ask friends who have successfully quit what worked for them. Some studies find that women tend to be more successful in small groups than large lecture settings. Check whether there are other women enrolled so you find others who understand what you're going through.

THE BOTTOM LINE

Be a quitter! If you smoke, there is nothing better that you can do for your health than quit. That is how monumentally the danger of smoking looms. If you've tried to quit before, don't give up. Most people who eventually succeed have failed before. For further help, consult the Resources section.

CHAPTER 16

STEP 2: EAT TO CONQUER THE ODDS

ONE OF YOUR BEST WEAPONS to conquer the odds is as close as your refrigerator. By wisely choosing the foods you eat, you may help protect yourself from several of the killer diseases outlined in this book, including heart disease, diabetes, and some types of cancer.

You may be surprised that this book does not contain a written-in-cement eating plan. That's because there isn't necessarily a right and wrong way to eat, as notes Sue Gebo, a registered dietitian in West Hartford, Connecticut, and author of the book *What's Left To Eat?* "No one meal plan meets everyone's needs. It really takes individual tailoring to make a plan work," she says.

When Gebo teaches her nutrition classes, she asks the participants how they make their eating choices. Their response? "They have about a million things that enter into it: taste, culture, economics, convenience, the time of preparation, you name it," she says.

It's not surprising, then, that restrictive food plans eventually fail. So do the plans outlined in diet books—even best-sellers—that pour onto the shelves each season. "Diet books are very restrictive. People get bored. People are well intentioned, but they stick to it for a couple of weeks, maybe a month at most," says Gebo.

The American Dieticians Association likes the government's

food pyramid, known as the Dietary Guidelines for Americans. Maybe it doesn't sound glamorous, but the recommendations are nutritionally sound and already paid for with your tax dollars.

You're probably familiar with this eating plan. It replaced the Four Basic Food Groups we grew up with. You can use the food pyramid as a broad base but create your own personally tailored eating plan, using the information in this chapter to help you conquer the odds.

How do you get the food pyramid plan? Just access the United States Agricultural Department's Food and Nutrition Center at http://www.nal.usda.gov/fnic/ or at the American Dietitians Association website at www.eat right.org. There is a wealth of nutritional information at both these websites as well.

Here's the basic menu for the food pyramid. The guidelines are designed for both men and women. Since most women require less food than men, use the lower number of suggested servings. The exception would be vegetables; you should eat at least five servings a day. Read on; you'll see why.

The reason this plan is called a food pyramid is the foods you should eat the most are on the bottom, and it continues upward to the foods you should eat the least, such as fats and oils. This plan also has the advantage in that it was used as the basis for the USDA's food labels, which are now on all processed foods. So as you scan your supermarket shelves, you'll find this handy reminder.

The best thing about this eating plan is that it enables you to eat anything you want—within moderation. That's important, because every day brings new myths and ill-advised edicts when it comes to food. For instance, I was recently at a picnic where lots of different foods were served, including a platter of thinly sliced rare roast beef. Moving down the line, one guest viewed this platter with disdain. In a tsk-tsk tone of voice, she observed to the hostess, "Well, that's not healthy." "Oh, I'm sorry," replied the hostess apologetically. She need not have apologized; the roast beef was an excellent source of protein as well as vitamin B_6, which has been getting attention lately as a possible fighter against heart disease. But so many negative comments have been made about red meat that there is a knee-jerk reaction against it.

That's true of any foods that contain fat, but not all fat is bad.

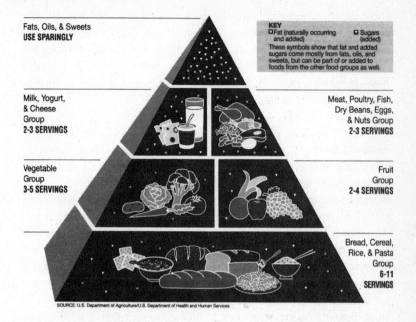

Fats, Oils, & Sweets
USE SPARINGLY

KEY
□ Fat (naturally occurring   ▪ Sugars
and added)   (added)
These symbols show that fat and added
sugars come mostly from fats, oils, and
sweets, but can be part of or added to
foods from the other food groups as well.

Milk, Yogurt,
& Cheese
Group
2-3 SERVINGS

Meat, Poultry, Fish,
Dry Beans, Eggs,
& Nuts Group
2-3 SERVINGS

Vegetable
Group
3-5 SERVINGS

Fruit
Group
2-4 SERVINGS

Bread, Cereal,
Rice, & Pasta
Group
**6-11
SERVINGS**

SOURCE: U.S. Department of Agriculture/U.S. Department of Health and Human Services

Mayonnaise, for instance, is shunned for its fat content, yet it is also rich in the antioxidant vitamin E.

Does this mean you should gorge on roast beef and mayonnaise sandwiches? No, but it does point out the wisdom of moderation.

If you wish, use this basic plan as your building blocks. Then use the information in the rest of this chapter to fill in your personalized eating plan based on your likes and dislikes. Make changes gradually to incorporate the foods and nutrients that can help you conquer the odds.

THE WEIGHT-LOSS DILEMMA

It's impossible to write about eating in a book for women without touching on the subject of dieting, because all too often what a woman chooses to eat is influenced by how she looks in the mirror rather than by nutrition. Three-quarters of American women have dieted in their lives, and at any given point in time up to one-half of us are on a diet. Our culture is obsessed with losing weight.

On the other hand, obesity is a risk factor for several of the killers listed in this book, including heart disease and diabetes. The answer "Lose weight" seems simple, but as most of us know (and the multibillion dollar diet industry shows), it's not.

For many of us (myself included), losing weight is a constant battle. This is because our weight is largely predetermined by our genetics. "Obesity is not directly inherited like height is, but you do inherit the tendency. You inherit a set of genes that make it difficult to maintain a certain weight," said Robert L. Jungas, Ph.D., professor of physiology in a lecture at the University of Connecticut Health Center's School of Medicine.

Studies show that identical twins have a 45 percent chance of both being too heavy, as compared to fraternal twins, who have a 5 percent chance of being heavy if the other is also overweight, he notes. On the other hand, findings show that we can modify this tendency. For instance, a child who is adopted into an overweight family usually becomes overweight, demonstrating that food habits are learned.

So although losing weight isn't easy, it can be done. Here are five principles that can help:

1. Diets Don't work

I went on my first diet at the age of 15, when the liquid diet Metrecal was in vogue, and I can still recall its chalky aftertaste. Back then Weight Watchers was just getting started; we handed around mimeographed sheets with recipes that used canned bean sprouts and tomato juice to make a poor facsimile of spaghetti and sauce.

There is always a new diet on the scene, and there are always plenty of women ready to try it. We've had the cabbage soup diet, the drinking man's diet, the fruit-only diet, the "It's not what you eat—it's when you eat it" diet. They all work—for a while. And eventually they all fail.

As Michael Fumento writes in his book The Fat of the Land, the first diet in book form was popularized more than a century ago, and they haven't stopped coming yet. According to Fumento, such diet books have these things in common:

- The authors are not experts, or if they are, their expertise is not in nutrition.
- Their diet promises weight loss without a change in habits or discipline.
- The food plan is too restrictive to stick to on a daily basis, year in, year out.

This is why, Fumento notes, "after more than thirty years of best-selling diet books, Americans are fatter than ever, and yet diet books continue to be best-sellers."

The most scientifically sound books—the ones written by authors with solid nutritional credentials—have these things in common:

- They advocate slow, gradual weight loss.
- They permit the eating of all foods in moderation.
- They recognize the need for discipline to change eating habits and exercise.

These diet plans are not fast or trendy, but they work.

2. Overcome Compulsive Eating/Dieting

That first liquid diet in the 1960s started me on a round of dieting that found me, twenty years later, still overweight. Furthermore, I was a compulsive eater, bingeing one day, dieting the next, and filled with self-loathing all the time. I'm not alone; because of our constant dieting and denial, many women are compulsive dieters—and compulsive eaters.

Not all women are compulsive eaters; many view food rationally and eat accordingly. If you are one of them, skip this section. If not, here are some questions to ask yourself to find out if you're a compulsive eater:

- Do words associated with food conjure up feelings of guilt and shame?
- Can you keep foods you like around without devouring them immediately?
- Do you constantly go on diets only to go off them just as quickly?
- Do you hate your body?
- Do your thoughts constantly revolve around food?

The key to overcoming compulsive eating is to give yourself permission to eat anything you want. Then, after you become accustomed to this, you can make healthy changes in your diet. This often sounds easier than it is. Books to help compulsive eaters can be found in the Resources section.

3. Self-Acceptance Is Key

Some women who diet unceasingly really are not too heavy at all. Obesity is defined as weighing 20 to 30 percent over your "ideal" body weight. But our medically "ideal" weight and the ideal image we carry with us in our minds can wildly differ.

"If you compare the size of a mannequin from 1950 to the present day, six inches have been lost from the hip. No wonder we all feel overweight," said Susan Calvert Finn, Ph.D., a registered dietitian who heads the American Dietetics Association's Nutrition and Health for Women Campaign at the third annual Congress on Women's Health in 1995. Accepting yourself as you are first is an important step toward breaking the yo-yo dieting pattern. But this is difficult.

In recent years the cult of thinness has been replaced by the cult of fitness, but the unrealistic images of models working out are often as unattainable as the images of supermodels, Nancy Clark, a registered dietitian in Brookline, Massachusetts, whose specialties include sports nutrition, wellness, and the management of eating disorders, said at the same conference. "Just leaf through the magazines, and you see women who are sleek, slender, strong, and slim. It's easy to get discouraged by these messages. Women throw up their hands," she says.

Happiness doesn't depend on the size of your jeans. Being good or bad are qualities related to your personal character, not the foods you eat or the size you wear. Even if we can lose weight, we may still have larger hips than we'd like. That shape is influenced by genetics and must be accepted. "Women, like fruit, come in differing sizes and shapes. We need to learn to honor that diversity," notes Nancy Clark.

4. Enjoy All Foods in Moderation

Just as you are not good or bad depending on the foods you eat, there are no good or bad foods. Consider chocolate, for instance. Renowned as a major female food craving, chocolate even made headlines in 1996 when astronaut Shannon Lucid, enroute to the Mir space station, sent back a request for M&Ms! That shouldn't be surprising. Chocolate is high in magnesium, which some women find helpful in dealing with hormonal symptoms around the time of their periods.

So it's not what you eat; it's how you balance these foods over the days, weeks, and months that makes the difference. The key to doing that is not a fancy formula or food lists; it's eating whatever you want to eat in moderation.

5. Exercise Is Essential

When you were growing up, you probably learned to count calories, not the miles you walked each day. But you'd have been better off tracking the miles. There's also evidence that it's a lack of fitness, not necessarily obesity, that raises the odds of many of the killer diseases. To create the best exercise program to conquer the odds, see the next chapter.

EATING TO BEAT YOUR RISK

While researching this book, I found the same general principles popping up over and over again. Use these principles to shape a healthy eating plan that can help you not only reduce the risk to specific diseases but also fashion a personal eating plan to be healthier in general.

1. Cut Back on Saturated Fat

In 1990, low-fat eating was all the rage, but now there is evidence that this enthusiasm has waned. Surveys have shown Americans returning to eating beef; steak restaurants are prospering; the makers of low-fat food lines like Snackwells are pumping out cookies and crackers that have some fat in them instead of the low-fat versions that were top sellers before. This more moderate view of fat is not a bad thing—many women went overboard before. But cutting back on fat—saturated fat especially—remains a worthwhile goal.

Saturated fat is believed to be a key component to raising the risk of heart disease. Eating a diet high in saturated fat can also lead to obesity, which contributes to diabetes. A diet high in saturated fat is linked to colon cancer and possibly others as well, including breast, skin, and ovarian cancer.

A Primer on Fat

All fats contain high amounts of calories, but they differ widely in their effects on our body. Generally, *saturated fat* raises blood cholesterol more than anything else you can eat. Examples of saturated fats include butter, lard, meat fat, shortening, and hydrogenated oils such as palm and coconut oil, palm kernel oil, and cocoa butter.

Trans-fatty acids have also been found to increase the risk of heart disease. These are found in margarine and also are a major ingredient in packaged baked goods, snack foods, and crackers. Unfortunately, this substance was not included in the most recent USDA food-labeling regulations, but there's a way to detect it. When you are looking at the label, add up all the types of listed fats; if your total falls short of the total fat listed on the label, the remaining amount is the amount of trans-fatty acids.

One of the cornerstones of a heart-healthy diet is to cut back on fat. According to the American Heart Association, we should obtain no more than 30 percent of our daily calories from fat, and only a third of that should come from saturated fat. Some experts believe this figure is too high and should be pared to 25 to 20 percent or even lower.

Is this the last word on fats? Not by a long shot. Our understanding of how certain fats are metabolized continues to grow. Remember when eggs were singled out as a cholesterol-raising villain? That's because egg yolks are composed of cholesterol. But it was found out later that eating them didn't necessarily translate into higher cholesterol levels in the body, especially if eaten in moderation. Some saturated fats once viewed as harmful, such as stearic acid, have been found to be less detrimental than was once believed. Foods containing this type of fatty acid include chocolate (yay!).

But just as with other areas of health, there is no firm agreement on every facet of nutrition, including the role of dietary fats and heart health.

The USDA's dietary guidelines call for the use of fats and oils only sparingly. But some experts believe that replacing saturated fats with monosaturated fats is helpful. A key proponent of this way of eating is Dr. Walter Willett, who heads the Nutrition Department of the Harvard School of Public Health. He favors a variation of the USDA food pyramid known as the traditional healthy Mediterranean diet pyramid. This diet is similar to the USDA food pyramid in that there is great emphasis on fruits, vegetables, and grains, and less on fish, poultry, and especially red meat. However, this plan allows for more fats than the USDA pyramid, as long as the fat is olive oil. (For more information, see *The Mediterranean Diet Cookbook*, listed in the Resources section.)

Some experts take issue with the notion that a low-fat diet is best for everyone. They contend that women who are insulin-resistant, which means their bodies overproduce insulin after eating sugar or starches, or those who have the trio of conditions known as syndrome X (diabetes, high triglycerides, and high LDL cholesterol) may be ill served by the much-touted low-fat diet.

This is because our bodies cannot distinguish between high-carbohydrate foods and sugar, so consuming a meal high in carbohydrates can result in overproduction of insulin, which is a hormone. In turn, the insulin can send the triglyceride level and the HDL cholesterol level down. For these women a moderate amount of fat in the diet is preferable to large amounts of carbohydrates.

His advice is aimed at women who have achieved their normal weight. Women who are overweight should lose weight by whatever method works for them, he believes.

These guidelines on fat will be much more refined in the future. Research is under way to identify more particular patterns of cholesterol and learn what type of diet can be used to achieve the best results.

If you want a more formal guide to losing weight by limiting your total fat intake, here's how to do it:

Figure out the number of calories a day you need to lose weight, and multiply it by the percentage of fat you should be eating in your daily diet. For instance, if you want only 20 percent of the food in your diet to come from fat, instead of the 35-40 percent that surveys show most adults eat, take the ideal number of calories you need to maintain your ideal weight (1,875, for example) and multiply that by 25 percent. That comes out to about 47 grams of fat a day. If you follow a 1,125 calorie a day plan, you would limit yourself to 28 grams of fat a day. You can eat a wide variety of foods, including a moderate amount of meat, as well as carbohydrate and protein, on such a plan. To make fat gram counting easier, pick up one of the fat gram counters on the market.

2. Replenish Calcium Daily and Take Vitamin D

As noted in chapter 13, calcium is vital for the functioning of our bodies. If your body runs out of the calcium it needs in your bloodstream, it is taken from the calcium stored in your bones. If too much is taken and not replaced, your bones can grow weak. So replenish your daily requirement of calcium by eating calcium-rich foods and taking calcium supplements. Both of these steps act together to ensure your body's calcium supply.

Calcium-Rich Foods

As a woman, it's very important to consume enough calcium. Unfortunately, most women think they can get away with just splashing some milk on their cereal. They're wrong. Studies find that although some women think they're getting enough calcium in their diet, they often fall short.

In recent years the government has increased the recommended amount of calcium for all women. The daily recommended levels for women are 1,000 mg for women before menopause and those on hormone replacement therapy, and 1,500 mg for women who are post menopause and not taking replacement hormones or are 65 years old or older. Women who are pregnant or breast-feeding should get 1,200 mg daily. Generally, studies find that women consume only 450 to 550 mg of calcium daily, about half what is needed.

Get as much calcium as you can from the food you eat. Dairy products are loaded with calcium. If you're concerned about fat, skim milk, nonfat and low-fat yogurt, and lower-fat cheeses have as much, if not more, calcium. Low-fat yogurt is also an excellent source of calcium.

Foods other than dairy products provide calcium as well. The list includes salmon, sardines, some bread and grain products, and certain vegetables. Broccoli, collard greens, and kale are all rich in calcium. With vegetables, let color be your guide: the darker they are, the more calcium they contain. The exception is spinach; it contains oxalates, which inhibits calcium absorption.

Add some calcium-rich soy foods, like tofu, to your diet. These will do your bones even more good if you eat them with the other Japanese staples, calcium-rich seaweed and sea greens.

Caffeine can block calcium absorption, so minimize the amount of black coffee you drink. Bear in mind that specialty coffees such as lattes deliver a hefty dose of calcium. Make sure yours is made with skim milk, so it doesn't deliver lots of unnecessary fat, too.

Beat Your Risk: Many women are lactose-intolerant, which means they lack the intestinal enzyme lactase that enables them to metabolize lactose, a sugar found in milk and other dairy products. If you have this problem, it certainly may inhibit your getting enough calcium. However, some studies find the people who are lactose-intolerant actually can tolerate small to moderate amounts of dairy products, especially if they are part of a meal.

You can also get lactase drops to help you digest these foods, or try lactose-reduced milk.

Calcium Supplements

Since studies have found that the usual intake of calcium falls well below the national recommendations, the National Institutes of Health recommends women take calcium supplements to compensate. Robert Heaney, M.D., professor of medicine at Creighton University, discussed this recommendation at the Third Annual Congress of Women's Health in 1995. He noted that the National Institutes of Health was very impressed with a study done in Lyons, France, which found that elderly women who took calcium supplements had fewer hip fractures. "This was a surprisingly rapid and gratifyingly large response to a relatively simple intervention," he said, adding that a mounting number of studies have similar findings.

Nonetheless, if you have significant bone loss or are at high risk for osteoporosis, calcium supplements won't take the place of estrogen or other osteoporosis medications. A study published in 1998 in the *Journal of Bone and Mineral Research*, which reported on a four-year study of 177 women between the ages of 61 and 70, found that those who took calcium supplements had less bone loss than the women who took a placebo, but the effect was much smaller than that of the other medications. However, if you are on those other bone-strengthening medications, getting enough calcium will enhance their effects.

Here are some tips for getting the most out of calcium supplements you take:

- Calcium supplements made from bone meal or crushed or fossilized oysters may contain high levels of lead or other toxic minerals. Because of this many experts recommend calcium carbonate.
- Avoid taking calcium with bulk-forming laxatives, which can reduce absorption.

- If you're taking an iron supplement as well, don't take it at the same time, since this can also block the absorption of calcium.

- Our bodies can absorb only about a 500 mg dose of calcium at a time, so take your supplements in small doses, spread throughout the day. Taking them at mealtime helps absorption.

Vitamin D

Although not as critical to bones as calcium, vitamin D is also important in the making of bone. We get most of this vitamin, aptly nicknamed the "sunshine vitamin," by absorbing it through our skin from the sun.

Traditionally, it was thought we got enough vitamin D from the sun. But that thinking has changed. A few years ago, after the government increased its daily recommendation for vitamin D from 200 to 400 international units (IU) for people aged 51 to 70 and 600 IU for those over 70, a study was published casting doubt on whether most people get this amount.

This study, published in 1998 in the *New England Journal of Medicine*, found that 57 percent of the participants had deficient levels of vitamin D. Although the study's participants were older hospitalized patients, the researchers noted that a separate analysis of young, healthy people had found that although their vitamin D levels were better, the problem was still widespread. These findings held true even for those people taking multivitamins.

Vitamin D plays a primary role in maintaining normal blood levels of calcium. If you are deficient in vitamin D, calcium is removed from the bone to make up the deficit, which can contribute to osteoporosis.

Our vitamin D supply can be too low because of inadequate exposure to sunlight. Ironically, the use of sunscreen, essential to ward off skin cancer, also inhibits the absorption of vitamin D. So make sure you're getting enough of this vitamin. Milk fortified with vitamin D, herring, salmon, mackerel, and tuna are sources.

Beat Your Risk: *Taking calcium supplements is not good for everyone. If you have kidney disease, get kidney stones, have chronic indigestion, or can't tolerate dairy products, ask your doctor what kind of calcium supplements you should use, if any.*

---

3. Eat Lots of Fruits and Vegetables

Eating at least five daily servings of both fruits and vegetables every day may lower the risk of cancer, coronary heart disease, and possibly stroke as well. Why? It's not known precisely, but they're loaded with antioxidant vitamins, including beta carotene (which the body converts to vitamin A), vitamin E, and vitamin C. In addition, there's evidence that fruits and vegetables contain scores of micronutrients that may protect against cancer.

Here's where to find them:

Vitamin C

Broccoli, brussels sprouts, cantaloupe, cauliflower, clams, currants (fresh), mangos, peppers, kiwis, papayas, oranges, parsley, pod peas, strawberries, red cabbages, grapefruit.

Vitamin E

Dried apricots, mangos, pumpkin seeds, fortified cereals, sweet potatoes, wheat germ, sunflower seeds, asparagus, raw kale.

Vitamin A and Beta Carotene

Broccoli, carrots, sweet potatoes, pumpkins, yellow squash, cooked spinach, tomatoes, kale, red peppers, red chili peppers, parsley, watercress, cantaloupe.

Fruits and vegetables also contain scores of micronutrients that may help protect against cancer and other diseases. Among them are the following:

Carotenoids. Beta carotene, an amino acid, is part of a family of chemicals known as carotenoids. People with a high level of beta carotene in their blood have been found to have a lower risk not only of cancer but also heart disease and stroke. It's believed that carotenoids contribute to the beneficial effect of beta carotene. Carotenoids are found in parsley, carrots, winter squash, sweet potatoes, yams, cantaloupe, apricots, spinach, kale, turnip greens, and citrus fruits.

Phytochemicals. Unlike vitamins, these chemicals have no nutritional value, but they are believed to be potent cancer fighters. For instance, broccoli, cauliflower, and brussels sprouts contain a chemical that has been demonstrated to block the growth of tumors in rats. Here are some examples of phytochemicals:

Flavonoids block receptor sites for certain hormones that promote cancer. Most fruits and vegetables contain flavonoids, including parsley, carrots, citrus fruits, broccoli, cabbage, cucumbers, squash, yams, eggplant, tomatoes, peppers, and berries. Soy products also contain them.

Indoles induce the formation of protective enzymes that may help fight cancer. They're found in cabbage, brussels sprouts, and kale.

These are major categories that are thought to help protect against cancer and other diseases. Most fruits and vegetables also contain scores of other chemicals that may also provide protection. These include *lycopene,* an antioxidant found in tomatoes and red grapefruit; *allylic sulfides,* contained in garlic and onions; and *linolenic acid,* found in many leafy vegetables and seeds, especially flaxseeds. But you don't have to turn your kitchen into a chemist's lab; be assured that if you're eating several servings of fruits and vegetables every day, you're consuming lots of these healthful substances.

4. Bulk Up on Fiber

You ordinarily wouldn't think that fiber, which is, after all, just the indigestible part of fruits, vegetables, and grains would deserve superstar status, but it does. Although it has no nutritional value in itself, fiber is credited with an impressive array of benefits.

A cholesterol fighter, fiber apparently helps lower the risk of coronary heart disease. Fiber is also credited with protecting against colon cancer, and it helps lower high blood pressure and improves the way diabetics metabolize sugar. Furthermore, fiber helps guard against gastrointestinal disorders such as irritable bowel syndrome. As a bonus, because foods rich in fiber stave off hunger, fiber is a boon to weight watchers.

Most experts recommend you try to eat 25 to 35 grams of fiber a day but don't go over 35. Since most processed foods don't contain any fiber, and foods rich in fiber contain only a few grams, it's difficult to reach that number anyway. Too much fiber too quickly can also upset your stomach; add it to your diet gradually, a few grams a day, and remember to drink plenty of water.

Foods rich in fiber are: most whole grains, oats, oat bran, oat flakes, rye crisp crackers, popcorn, toasted wheat germ, granola, high-fiber bread, and all types of beans; also many fruits, including apples, figs, peaches, pears, prunes, raspberries, and strawberries, as well as many types of vegetables, including asparagus, beets, broccoli, carrots, kale, corn, okra, potatoes with skin, and zucchini.

Here are some tips for getting more fiber in your diet:

- Clean fruits and vegetables, but leave the peels on.
- Use oats as a filler in casseroles or meat loaf.
- Use whole grains when you bake.
- Snack on raw fruits and vegetables, air-popped popcorn, or low-fat cereal mix instead of high-fat, low-fiber chips.
- Read bread labels carefully. Some whole-grain breads are rich in fiber, but many that are labeled "whole grain" or "whole wheat" have no more fiber than white bread.

5. Learn the Joy of Soy Foods

If you're of Asian descent or a vegetarian, you're probably familiar with soy foods. There's increasing evidence that soy, a substance made from soybeans, may lower the risk of a host of diseases, including heart disease, because it lowers cholesterol; breast cancer, because it contains phytoestrogen, a substance that chemically resembles estrogen and may block cancer-promoting receptor cells in the breast; and osteoporosis, because it is rich in calcium.

Dr. Susan Love, the breast cancer expert, is an enthusiastic soy advocate. "I eat soy every day, absolutely. I have nonfat soy milk with my cereal, miso soup for lunch, some tofu here and there," says Dr. Love.

How do you incorporate soy into your diet? It's easier than ever, with soy products making their way into the supermarket, disguised as more familiar foods, for example, soy burgers. Tofu, though bland in itself, is spongy and soaks up flavor, so it can pitch-hit for chicken or beef in stir-fried dishes, for example. Other soy products include tempeh, a thin cake made from fermented soybeans, isolate soy protein, soy flour, soya powder, textured soy powder, and soy milk.

Beat Your Risk: *Although soy can be considered a health food, beware of soy sauce. It has some nutritional value, but it is very high in salt. Also, when it is used to make teriyaki sauce, sugar is added.*

---

6. Indulge in Alcohol Moderately

Since a few years ago when the television show *60 Minutes* publicized the concept known as "the French paradox," the health benefits of alcohol have been a hot topic. The French paradox refers to the fact that the French traditionally eat a rich diet, yet they have one of the lowest rates of heart disease in the industrialized world. How can this be so? One possible explanation is that the French drink wine with their meals.

More than a dozen studies have found that the moderate consumption of alcoholic beverages—be it wine, beer, or liquor—reduces heart disease risk by 35 to 50 percent. Evidence suggests that much of this benefit is due to the fact that alcohol increases the amount of HDL (good) cholesterol in the blood. There's also evidence that alcohol may favorably affect blood clotting, reducing the risk of heart attack. These protective effects are found whether wine, beer, or alcohol is consumed. However, red wine and dark beer also may have antioxidant effects that can help retard the effects of aging on the heart's vessels. By the way, teetotalers can get this beneficial effect by drinking grape juice.

However, before you imbibe, there are other factors to take into account. First, the studies show that these protective effects are true only for those who indulge moderately; for women, this is defined as one drink—a standard drink being 12 ounces of beer, 4 ounces of wine, or 1.5 ounces of 80-proof spirits.

In contrast, studies find that women who drink heavily are more likely than men to develop such serious health problems as cardiomyopathy—a disease that destroys the heart muscle—and potentially deadly liver diseases, like cirrhosis and hepatitis. Female heavy drinkers are also believed to be more prone to alcoholism, depression, and suicide.

As for whether drinking alcohol protects against stroke, the evidence is contradictory. For ischemic strokes, the type caused by narrow or blocked arteries, light drinkers are at less risk than nondrinkers, but those who indulge too much are at far higher risk. For hemorrhagic stroke, it's a different story. A Finnish study reported in 1993 in the journal *Stroke* found that women who had drunk large amounts of alcohol suffered more strokes. But the total effect of alcohol is difficult to sort out, because these drinkers may also have taken drugs such as cocaine, or amphetamines, which also cause stroke.

There is also concern that alcohol drinkers raise their risk of breast cancer. Studies have linked heavy drinking to this ailment, and a few also have pointed to moderate amounts as problematic. A study published in 1995 in the *Journal of the National Cancer Institute* found that women who drank as few as one and a half drinks per day increased their risk of breast cancer. The risk went up the more they drank. According to this particular study, wine consumption did not increase breast cancer risk, but the researchers refused to let wine drinkers off the hook, citing other studies that show increased risk. But this may still be undetermined, because some studies put moderate and heavy drinkers in one group.

It's not known why consuming alcohol might increase the risk of breast cancer, but research has demonstrated that when women drink alcohol at certain times during their menstrual cycles, their levels of several hormones increase. More study is needed to confirm this and also link it to breast cancer.

So if you are looking to your health as an excuse to start drinking, you won't find it here. On the other hand, drinking lightly, or in moderation, may offer some health benefits.

Beat Your Risk: *Studies repeatedly show that Americans don't drink enough water. Eight glasses a day is the recommendation. Caffeinated substances like tea and coffee don't count; they can actually be dehydrating. So keep a water bottle with you.*

WHAT ABOUT SUPPLEMENTS?

It's amazing how many people distrust doctors, but are willing to down handfuls of vitamins and supplements on the recommendation of their neighbor, hairdresser, or even the guy on television doing an infomercial. "Indeed, it often seems that people usually will trust anyone except their doctor or a trained dietitian," notes Sue Gebo.

This faith in the value of vitamins and nutritional supplements fuels an enormously successful industry. In 1993 it was estimated that Americans spent $4 billion on 3,400 different nutritional products. Since then the industry has steadily grown.

Do you need to take vitamin and mineral supplements to conquer the odds? As long as you're eating a healthy diet, the answer, generally, is no, says the American Dietetic Association (ADA). Although vitamins and minerals certainly are very important, they're most beneficial when you get them when they are part of foods, the organization contends.

In its position paper on vitamin supplements, the ADA found increased interest in determining which nutrients optimize health and whether these can be adequately obtained from your diet or must be supplemented. In particular, the organization notes studies which find that eating lots of fruits and vegetables helps prevent cancer. There's also increased interest in the role of antioxidants, including beta carotene, vitamin C, and vitamin E, in the prevention of heart disease.

The ADA contends that the best nutritional strategy for both good health and disease prevention is to obtain those nutrients from a wide variety of foods. Supplements are appropriate "when well-accepted, peer-reviewed, scientific evidence shows safety and effectiveness," the ADA notes.

Although it is true that the majority of Americans use supplements, this doesn't change the evidence that they don't do as good a job as eating whole foods. Want some proof?

First, much remains unknown about the biologically active compounds in food and how they impact on the body. There are numerous compounds in foods that are not essential nutrients but have properties which show they may help prevent heart disease and cancer. Consider the study on smokers and vitamin supplements cited in chapter 8. This study found that smokers with high levels of beta carotene, which is found in fruits and vegetables, in their blood had a lower lung cancer risk. But when the study's participants were given this vitamin in supplement form, their lung cancer rate actually increased.

Although other studies of the benefits of vitamin supplements have sometimes made headlines, what is sometimes missed is that these were studies done in people who were eating a poor diet to begin with. For instance, a study published in 1993 in the *Journal of the National Cancer Institute* found that giving vitamins to inhabitants of Linxian, China, helped prevent death from esophageal cancer, which occurs at a high rate there. However, the people in this study were drawn from a region that has a nutritionally deficient diet, so it's not known if people living in America would realize the same benefit.

How can you make decisions on supplements? The same principles as reading medical studies on other topics, discussed earlier in
this book, apply. To recap:

- Don't rely on any single study or news article; give most credence to those that draw their conclusion from much research.
- Pay the most attention to research that's published in scientific, peer-reviewed journals.
- Pay attention to recommendations from such organizations
as the American Heart Association, the American Cancer Society, and the National Institutes of Health, which make their recommendation after considerable debate and study.
- Be aware that since research is always ongoing, these recommendations are subject to revision.

The government is constantly updating its nutritional recommendations. Here are the latest findings on supplements that have
proved to be valuable:

Folate (known also as folic acid): It's now recommended that
adults consume 400 micrograms daily and that pregnant women and
those planning to become pregnant consume 600 micrograms. Research shows that folate deficiency in pregnant women can cause
neural-tube defects, such as spina bifida, in infants. Folate also lowers
homocysteine, the amino acid that may play a role in heart disease.
Ideally, you should obtain folate from food; it occurs naturally in
spinach, beans, nuts, and citrus fruits. Bread, cereal, pasta, and other
grains are now also being fortified with it. But if you plan to become
pregnant, or you are pregnant, and you don't consume enough of it,
a supplement is recommended.

Calcium and vitamin D: Current recommendations are noted earlier in this chapter. The daily recommended levels for women are
1,000 mg for women before menopause and 1,500 mg thereafter. For
vitamin D, 400 IU for anyone age 51 and older; 600 IU for anyone
71 and older.

Regarding *multivitamins*, the American Dietetic Association does
not deem them necessary unless you are:

- A strict vegetarian who doesn't consume any animal products
- On a very low-calorie weight-loss diet
- Elderly and not eating as much as you used to and should
- Aware that you don't eat a healthy diet

SUPPLEMENTS YOU SHOULD CONSIDER: THE ANTIOXIDANTS

Although there isn't complete evidence of it, vitamin E and the other antioxidants show promise in preventing heart disease.

Vitamin E has received the most media attention. A survey from the Nurses' Health Study, published in 1993 in the *New England Journal of Medicine*, found that women taking vitamin E supplements for more than two years reduced their heart disease risk by 40 percent. Other studies find similar results.

It's not known exactly why vitamin E may be protective, but the hypothesis is that oxidation, a process that occurs in our body's cells with every breath we take, may contribute to heart disease. Vitamin E and other antioxidants are believed to block this process.

Taking vitamin E supplements is popular because you can't consume it naturally in the quantities used in the research studies. But you can obtain at least some vitamin E from the food you eat. A study published in 1996 in the *New England Journal of Medicine* showed that this may prove beneficial. Researchers queried 34,486 women and found that those who ate foods containing vitamin E— specifically nuts, margarine, and mayonnaise—had a lower risk of dying of heart disease. Bear in mind, though, that although the headlines portrayed this as "It's okay to eat fatty food after all," the study was not a wholesale endorsement of pigging out on cheeseburgers. Indeed, the women who ate the most foods with natural vitamin E still ate relatively modest amounts of fatty foods, such as salad dressing made with mayonnaise. Another endorsement of moderation!

Another set of nutrients being explored are the B vitamins, including folic acid, because of their effect on homocysteine, the amino acid that may contribute to heart disease. More research is needed before these supplements are recommended, but fruits and vegetables are high in folic acid, and you should be eating a lot of them anyway.

Since the scientific proof for the claims made for many vitamins and supplements doesn't exist, you may wonder why the manufacturers are allowed to make health claims. The answer lies in the Dietary Supplement Health and Education Act of 1994. The passage of that law granted makers of dietary supplements and herbal preparations greater freedom to make these claims. You can identify these products by the fact that they bear the required disclaimer stating that the claim has not been evaluated by the FDA.

Just because a supplement is sold in a health food store or labeled "natural," that doesn't necessarily mean it is harmless. Here are a few examples of the dangers of vitamin overuse: too much vitamin A can cause birth defects if taken by pregnant women; too much calcium can limit the absorption of iron; and too much zinc can impair the immune response and negatively affect cholesterol levels. If you're uncertain about a supplement you're tempted to take, or if you're considering megadoses, check with your doctor.

EATING TIPS TO REDUCE YOUR RISK

This book does not contain a specific eating "plan" because, in the long run, such plans don't work. You are the best judge of what you wish to eat. On the other hand, you can use these strategies to tailor your own healthy meals. Feel free to think up your own. (If you'd like to share them, you can e-mail them to me at char@libov.com, and I'll post them on the Women's Health Hot Line website at www.libov.com.)

1. Viva Variety

Choose your foods from a wide variety of categories, making sure you eat plenty of fruits, vegetables, and fiber daily. Don't necessarily rule out any food as a no-no; lean meat is fine in moderation, as are fats, when they are used sparingly, and even a piece of chocolate is okay now and then.

2. Let Color Be Your Guide

Color is a guide you can use to add variety to your meals. What's pleasing to the eye is often nutritious as well, and if you vary the colors of your food, you'll be getting a mix of vitamins. Make a colorful mix of red and yellow peppers; add purple eggplant. Leave potatoes in their crinkly, brown, full-of-fiber jackets. Fix a gorgeous fruit bowl. Tempt your eye as well as your palate.

3. Eat Your Protein "on the Side"

In the old days, the day's protein choice—meat, poultry, or fish—was considered the main dish, with the vegetables going "on the side." Nowadays, we know that although protein is important, less is best. So double up on the veggies and enjoy a three-ounce serving of protein "on the side."

4. Make Smart Substitutions

Thanks to the emphasis on low-fat eating, there are now lots of low-fat substitutes for foods that were formerly high in fat. Not everybody likes the "no fat" versions; you may find the "reduced fat" items tastier and more satisfying. For instance, top a grilled vegetable patty (made from healthful soy) with reduced-fat cheese or a smaller serving of genuine cheese. Want some bacon with that? Try turkey bacon. Mix and match any way you please. But beware of fat-free baked goods; if you start eating fat-free desserts when you didn't before, the calories can quickly mount up. Also, sometimes when fat is removed, sugar is added.

5. Eat Your Meals When You Want

Despite the claims of best-selling diet books, there's no evidence that adhering to a certain dining schedule is better than another, or that combining foods makes any difference. It's your total daily eating that counts. Some folks prefer to eat two or three large meals a day; others like to spread their total intake into several smaller meals. Do whichever you prefer. If you're not cooking only for yourself, compromise may be in order. For instance, if you find you're hungriest at lunch, you can still eat your larger meal then and eat more lightly at dinner with your family.

6. Learn the Joy of Soy

Soy is a health bonanza; it lowers cholesterol, and it is loaded with calcium, as well as substances that may reduce breast cancer risk and ease menopausal symptoms like hot flashes. Vegetarian and Japanese cookbooks can guide you in how to use soy, and you'll also find recipes in *Super Soy: The Miracle Bean* and *The Soy Gourmet*, two books listed in the Resources section.

7. Eat and Take Out Wisely

Restaurants and takeout businesses are skyrocketing as fewer of us cook. You don't need to forgo eating out; just make wise choices. Here are some strategies:

- If you're a light eater, consider ordering an appetizer instead of an entree.
- If you've chosen a dish such as French onion soup, which is covered in baked cheese, ask the kitchen to hold the cheese, or if you don't want to do that, request a lesser amount. You can sometimes do this for takeout dishes as well.
- Don't go famished. If you're planning to go out to eat at six-thirty, remember that it may be seven-thirty before your meal actually arrives. Have some yogurt or fruit late in the afternoon so you're not tempted to devour the bread basket.
- If the restaurant you go to makes large portions, ask that half of it be wrapped up as a doggie bag before the dish is even brought to the table; that way you won't be tempted to eat more than you want.
- Be careful about liquor. If you drink throughout your meal,

you may end up drinking a good portion of calories; plus, those drinks may put you in a frame of mind that makes conscious eating difficult.

• Don't be shy; ask if a dish can be made with a noncreamy sauce or if you can substitute a baked potato for French fries. It doesn't hurt to ask, and many restaurants like to be accommodating.

8. Be Uneconomical

Dinners that come with free sundaes, "super size" specials offering giant-sized meals and fries at cheap rates, and penalty charges for shared meals can make eating wisely cost more. Manufacturer's coupons are usually for processed foods, not fruits and vegetables. Driving to the supermarket with the freshest produce may cost more, and that out-of-season container of raspberries can be much pricier than a candy bar. But remember, eating wisely pays big dividends, and you're worth it.

9. Give Yourself Time

If at five minutes to six you're just starting to think about what you're going to eat for dinner, you probably won't be eating a well-balanced meal. It may take a little more time to learn to eat wisely in the beginning; you need to learn what you want to have on hand, find some appealing recipes, and decide what you really do like to eat. Taking the extra time is worth it; you'll be building good habits that will serve you well for years.

10. Make Changes Gradually

It's very tempting to make dramatic changes in one's diet, and then sit back and wait for the miraculous results. When they don't happen, we get frustrated, and the diet goes into the trash can. Instead, start gradually. Switch to a bagel with reduced-fat cream cheese instead of a higher-fat muffin, 2 percent milk instead of whole, a fruit salad topped with yogurt instead of ice cream. Before you know it, these changes will become healthy habits.

THE BOTTOM LINE

No magic food has been found that will guarantee you will conquer the odds, but fruits and vegetables come the closest. Fiber is good, and soy may be the miracle food of the future. In terms of losing weight, low-fat diets work for many, but they're not a foolproof solution for everyone. Cutting back on calories and exercising may not be glamorous, but it's the best way to trim down and keep the weight off. There are no "good" foods and "bad" foods, and that includes chocolate!

17

STEP 3: GET MOVING!

The lights dim, and Lauretta Caron steps onto the stage. She spins across the floor, swirling her colorful veils, her spangles glittering under the lights. Her audience bursts into applause. At age 70, Lauretta shows no sign of slowing down. She's a belly dancer, and she means to keep it up.

What's Lauretta's secret? In a newspaper interview, she gave credit to exercise. She rises at dawn every morning and performs 80 push-ups and 80 sit-ups, a regimen many of us younger women would find daunting. Lauretta is a believer in the magic of exercise. Unfortunately, most of us are not. In fact, only 27 percent of American women exercise regularly, according to government statistics.

Even worse, the older we get, the more we need to exercise. Yet as we age, the less we do. Why don't we exercise? There are plenty of reasons.

"Many older women believe that exercise is a bad thing, that it's inappropriate, and they should act their age," said Martha Storandt, Ph.D., in an interview regarding a study she headed on exercise attitudes published in 1996 in the journal *Health Psychology*.

Although lack of activity is a problem that cuts across all races and ethnic groups, African-Americans and minority women exercise less than white women, says Shiriki Kumanyika, Ph.D., director of the Department of Human Nutrition and Dietetics at the University of Illinois at Chicago. She discovered that African-Americans don't realize that exercise benefits health; they think it would just add one more stress on their already stressful lives. Socioeconomic factors take their toll as well; many single parents said they had too many family responsibilities. Health clubs are expensive, and unsafe neighborhoods make being outdoors dangerous.

Some women tell me they are reluctant to go to health clubs because they don't want to wear leotards or bathing suits in public. Or they don't feel coordinated enough to try an aerobics class, or they're simply afraid they're too old. But the number one reason most women give is that they simply don't have time.

We shouldn't feel this way. Exercise is very important—possibly the most important health behavior we can have.

At the Copper Institute for Aerobics Research in Dallas Texas, many leading studies are done on the health aspects of exercise. Steven Blair, P.E.D., director of research there, has found that people who are not physically fit are at a higher risk of dying earlier. It doesn't make a difference whether they're fat or trim, he has said in written interviews.

We must revamp our attitudes. Study after study hails the healthful effects of exercise. Experts estimate that as many as 250,000 deaths per year in the United States can be attributed to a lack of regular exercise.

As noted in earlier chapters of this book, exercise reduces the risk of a host of diseases that kill women. Here's a summary:

Breast Cancer. Women who regularly exercise in their younger years reduce their breast cancer risk by an estimated 30 to 60 percent, and there's evidence that older female exercisers benefit as well.

Colon cancer. Over the past 20 years, studies have found that women who exercise regularly have lower colon cancer rates, possibly because exercise promotes efficient digestion and elimination.

Diabetes. When you exercise, your body uses insulin more efficiently, greatly reducing the risk of diabetes.

Heart disease. Several studies find that regular exercise can lower a woman's risk of heart disease, no matter what her age, by about 40 percent or even more.

Osteoporosis. Exercise is one of the most efficient ways to build up bone mass, no matter what a woman's age.

Stroke. Just as regular exercise reduces a woman's risk for heart disease, it does so for stroke.

If exercise only afforded these benefits, that would be plenty of reason to do it. But there are a host of additional advantages, notes Rita Watson, M.P.H., an author who writes about stress. "Exercise has been shown to reduce anxiety and stress, improve memory, and increase a sense of well-being. As if that's not enough, aerobic exercise seems to enhance creativity, quite independently of its effect on mood," she says. She acknowledges that it isn't known why exercise has such positive effects, but she adds, "Theories include regaining control of one's body, altering chemical substances in the brain, or elevating body temperature, which could have an effect on the brain."

Exercise also:

- Helps you lose weight and keep it off
- Reduces high blood pressure
- Tones your muscles
- Helps you think more clearly
- Helps you sleep
- Reduces stress
- Alleviates depression
- Enhances your self-esteem

By the way, becoming physically fit does not mean you need to become a superwoman. It means you can accomplish such everyday activities as raking leaves, taking brisk walks, or playing with your kids (and later, your grandkids), and you can maintain this level of conditioning throughout your life.

THE THREE TYPES OF EXERCISE WOMEN NEED

Exercise is a tremendous boon for both men and women, but women have special needs. In fact, we need three different types of exercise for optimum fitness, as follows. Don't get discouraged—this is a good thing, since it builds variety into your routine.

Aerobic Exercise (for Endurance)

This is a continuous form of exercise in which your body meets your muscles' increased demand for oxygen. It improves the functioning of your cardiovascular system, including your heart. Aerobic exercise builds endurance as well.

It used to be thought that to be beneficial, aerobic exercise must be performed for at least a 20-minute period three times a week. But you can also derive benefits from doing it for shorter periods of time, such as 10 minutes at the start and end of each day, for example.

Examples of aerobic activities include: brisk walking, jogging, race walking, swimming, pool aerobics, bicycling (either stationary or on a real bicycle), aerobic dancing, folk dancing, calisthenics, using rowing and skiing machines, and using free weights and pulleys.

Anaerobic Exercise (for Strength)

Last November I received a call from my mother. "Is Terry going to be home for Thanksgiving dinner?" she asked. "Yes," I replied, "why?" "Well, Aunt Zelda made a fruit salad, but it's too heavy to carry from the car, so I was hoping he would help," my mother said.

My mother wasn't joking. Yes, the ceramic bowl was a little on the heavy side, but the idea that a man was needed to carry it into the house was quite sad—though not surprising. As we age, women lose strength in their upper arms so gradually that it can slip away without being noticed. But we need that upper-arm strength—to carry bundles, to lift our grandchildren, and yes, even to carry in the fruit salad.

The idea of women building up muscles once seemed odd, but no longer. Indeed, studies are finding that such training can dramatically offset the effects of aging. Such exercise is called *anaerobic*, which means that it is strenuous activity in which oxygen is used faster than the blood can supply it.

For novices, experts recommend using weight machines, such as Nautilus, because they put out even resistance, and limit the range of motion, and beginners are less apt to make mistakes or hurt themselves on them. But with proper instruction, you can achieve effective results using free weights.

Nowadays, the "buffed" look has become quite desirable for younger women. Older women may worry about becoming too muscular. Don't fret. Working with weights will give you a stronger, firmer body, but unless you perform lengthy workouts daily, you won't end up looking muscle-bound.

Beat Your Risk: *If you're doing aerobic activity too strenuously, your body can run out of oxygen that your muscles need and begin working anaerobically. This isn't desirable; it means your body is working too hard. To check yourself, use the talk test. If you can talk aloud while you perform aerobic exercise, you're working at the correct pace.*

Weight-Bearing Exercise (to Prevent Osteoporosis)

Weight-bearing exercises involve impact on the joints and, in doing so, stimulate the ends of your bones. There are two ways to build these into your activities. One is by choosing aerobic activities that apply some force to the bones; walking, jogging, aerobic dancing, and racquet sports all qualify as both aerobic and weight-bearing activities. One of the best exercises, which combines both aerobic and weight-bearing exercise, is to walk briskly and swing your arms. Even the most sophisticated exercise equipment can't beat it.

FAQS (FREQUENTLY ASKED QUESTIONS) ABOUT EXERCISE

Q. I spend a lot of time on my feet just doing my daily activities at work and at home. Isn't that enough?

A. No. To get the most out of exercise, your activity should not be related to the type of work you normally do. If you're chasing after the dog, picking up after your youngsters, or trotting from meetings to power lunch, your mind is on the task at hand, not on exercising your body.

Q. How much exercise do I need?

A. Although we don't put it this way, what most of us mean with that question is: "How little exercise can I get away with?" A general recommendation is to exercise three to five times per week at a level strenuous enough to raise your heart rate to a moderate level, and do two sessions per week of muscle-strengthening exercises.

Q: I'm confused. Some articles I've read say that the only exercise that counts is vigorous activity. Others say exercise that is not as intense still has benefits. What's the truth?

A: Actually there's some truth in both these views. The debate started when the Centers for Disease Control and the American College of Sports Medicine issued a joint statement urging Americans to perform 30 minutes of moderate activity every day. This exercise could be done all at once or accumulated throughout the day. Furthermore, the exercising didn't have to be strenuous; activities like gardening, raking leaves, and dancing counted. This was a departure from the government's previous stance, which recommended daily, sustained, vigorous activity.

Several months later, though, a study in the *New England Journal of Medicine* reported that women runners, whose exercise levels far exceeded these revised guidelines, benefited much more than less active women. That these two findings contradicted each other was widely broadcast.

What is right? It all depends on how active you ordinarily are.

The Center for Disease Control's "kinder, gentler" exercise guidelines were intended to encourage millions of Americans who are inactive to change their ways, not to tell those who are active to slack off. So if you're active already, stick with, or consider even stepping up, your current program. But if you don't exercise at all, or you do so only occasionally, the milder guidelines are more realistic. Ease into them and gradually increase your activity level.

Q: Getting started on an exercise program isn't my problem; sticking to it is. Any suggestions?

A: You're not alone. It's estimated that half of us who begin an exercise program give it up within six months. Fitness expert Joan Price, author of *Joan Price Says, Yes, You CAN Get in Shape,* specializes in motivating nonexercisers. "Whatever gets you moving and using your muscles counts as exercise, whether it's walking the dog, mowing the lawn, dancing, hiking, or playing ball with the kids. Chose an activity that will make exercise a treat," she advises in her book.

One way to find a fitness activity that appeals to you is to recall what you enjoyed doing when you were young, then update it. For instance, if you enjoyed roller skating as a kid, try inline skating. If you loved to dance, try ballroom or Western-style dancing. If you loved to swim, try a water aerobics class.

For more tips on getting started—and staying motivated—see the next section.

Q: What if I'm over 55?

A: If you're over 55, your body needs exercise as much, or even more, than if you're younger. Just ask Dr. Joel Posner, chief of geriatrics and rehabilitation medicine at the Medical College of Pennsylvania. "We believe a vigorous program of exercise is necessary for all people, particularly women from 55 years old on. I'm not talking about walking, I'm not talking about gardening, I'm not talking about playing with your grandchildren. I'm talking about training," he told doctors at the Third Annual Congress on Women's Health in Washington, D.C., in 1995. "Training for old age is as difficult as training for a decathlon in the Olympics," he added.

Q: What if I'm 65 or older?

A: If you're over 65, the idea of muscle building might strike you as quite odd. But there's evidence that everyone can benefit from this form of exercise, no matter what their age. A study published in 1994 in the *New England Journal of Medicine* found that a group of nursing home patients who received weight training improved their leg strength and mobility; some of the participants were even able to exchange their walkers for canes. Exercise experts Michael Pollock, Ph.D., and William F. Brechue, Ph.D., of the University of Florida's Center for Exercise Science, agree that no one is ever too old to exercise. Here are their recommendations for older women.

- Minimize the possibility of injury by choosing low-impact activities instead of high-impact ones. Low-impact activities include walking, biking, swimming, rowing, cross-country skiing, stair climbing, step aerobics, and low-impact aerobics.
- You can reap the same cardiovascular benefits from exercising at a lower intensity longer, as opposed to a shorter, more vigorous workout.
- Shoot for slow and steady progress. When you're over 65, it takes longer to gradually increase the intensity of your workout.
- If you have physical limitations, such as poor vision, an unsteady gait, or musculoskeletal limitations, don't be deterred. Instead, work with your doctor to find the most appropriate activities.

Beat Your Risk: *Your doctor should applaud your willingness to exercise. If your doctor is unenthusiastic, find out why. If there are medical considerations, discuss which type of activities would be good for you. But if your doctor seems to believe in the myth that exercise is inappropriate for older people, you might consider finding another doctor.*

Q: What if I have arthritis?

A: Exercise. Fifty years ago, doctors cautioned their patients with arthritis against exercise. Then it became apparent that physical inactivity leads to bone and muscle loss, so today people with arthritis are taught to exercise to keep their affected joints in as good working order as possible and to do conditioning exercises to promote fitness. This is important; researchers find that arthritis patients are more likely to develop heart disease, apparently because of their inactivity. But if you have arthritis, you need to work with your doctor or physical therapist to create the best program.

Beat Your Risk: *If you are over 55 and have a heart problem, diabetes, high blood pressure, or other major risk factors for heart disease, starting or intensifying an exercise program may trigger a heart attack. If this applies to you, or if you have any doubt about your ability to safely exercise, seek your doctor's advice. On the other hand, don't let this recommendation discourage you. Even a simple 10-minute daily walk can get you started on a healthier lifestyle.*

EXERCISE STRATEGIES FOR REDUCING YOUR RISK

You may notice that this book doesn't contain a specific exercise plan, just as it doesn't contain a diet plan. The reason is the same— plenty of books and magazines offer exercise plans, and people begin them with great enthusiasm. But six months later, or even sooner, they are only memories. No one knows your schedule, your preferences, and your level of fitness better than you do. By using the following strategies, you can build a more active lifestyle that will help you conquer the odds. (Do you have other strategies that you want to share? E-mail them to me at char@ibov.com so I can share them in my Women's Health Hot Line website at www.libov.com.)

1. Make an Exercise Appointment

A study performed for the President's Council on Physical Fitness and Sports found that not having enough time was the number one reason respondents gave for not exercising. This does not surprise me. When I give my health presentations, many women tell me that they don't have the time to exercise. They say to me, "'I'm the caregiver. I can't take the time away from my kids." Well, you need to include someone else in that picture, which is yourself. You need to take care of yourself.

Find a win-win solution. For example, if you're dropping off your kids at karate and you have an hour before you pick them up, go to a park and take a walk. Draw up a schedule and mark off the times you have to exercise.

You can also combat this problem by making a specific appointment for exercise—write it in your appointment book if you need to. If you're a morning person, do your exercise when you first get up. If you're a night person, you might want to schedule it later in the day.

2. Find a Buddy—or Exercise Alone If You Prefer

Some of us prefer to exercise alone; others like to find a buddy. Find the style that fits you best. I prefer to go on a walk with a friend; our conversation makes the time fly. But my neighbor prefers to power walk alone; she says that talking breaks her concentration. It's your exercise plan—it's your preference.

3. Exercise at Home or Join a Health Club

Again, it's up to you. Too often people sign up for an expensive health club contract, go a lot during the first few weeks, and then stop because they're bored, they've overdone it, or their needs are not being met. If you decide to join a health club, here are some questions to ask yourself:

- How convenient is the facility to you?
- Are the exercise times good for your schedule?
- Is the facility clean and well maintained?
- Are exercise classes too crowded?
- Is there a long wait to use equipment?
- Does the facility offer a variety of equipment?

Many people join health clubs to take advantage of the schedule of exercise classes offered. The class, though, is only as good as its leader. Ask to meet the staff and participate in a trial workout.

It's important to feel comfortable at a health club. Some women enjoy the fast pace of a club that caters to younger people; others, who want to bring the kids, might prefer a more family-oriented center, like a Y or a Jewish community center.

Look before you leap, financially. Read any contract carefully before you join. Check with your local Better Business Bureau and state consumer protection division to find out if any complaints have been filed against the club you are considering.

Often colleges and hotels have excellent physical fitness facilities, which they may allow the public to use for a fee that is sometimes less than a health club membership. If you live in the area where you attended college, your alumni status may enable you to use your alma mater's facilities free or at a reduced rate.

You don't need to join a health club to get fit, though. Many women prefer to exercise in their homes. There are many fitness shows on television. With VCRs it is easier now to exercise at home than ever before. There is a wide variety of exercise videos designed for women of all ages, fitness ability, and musical tastes. You may even be able to try them out by borrowing them from your local library or renting them from a video store.

4. Dress for (Exercise) Success

Exercise garb is a serious issue for many of us. We feel self-conscious about our bodies at a health club or even outdoors. If you don't like yourself in a leotard, opt for a colorful oversized T-shirt. There are some attractive exercise ensembles that come in larger sizes. Choose an exercise class where the women come in all ages and sizes—just like life!

5. Learn to Sweat!

Many older women are not comfortable sweating or are scared to exercise to the extent that they sweat. If that's how you feel, consider hiring a fitness trainer to teach you how to exert yourself safely. "One of the most rewarding aspects of this job is when I see someone who was just going through the motions really attacking the stationary bike. Something just clicked, and they've gotten into it," says Joy Kistler.

6. Don't Call It Exercise—Call It Fun!

Betsy, a 53-year-old librarian, recently went to a ballroom dancing class as a lark, but before she knew it, "I was hooked," she says. Recently she competed in her first ballroom dance competition—in black chiffon, no less. A picture of her and her instructor doing the tango is now one of her favorite possessions.

If you aren't interested in organized exercise, find an activity that's fun for you. Options include starting a walking club with your friends, going dancing, or getting involved with a sport. You don't need to call it exercise, you can call it fun.

7. Walk, Walk, Walk!

A brisk walk three times a week can afford the type of cardiovascular benefits once associated with more strenuous activities like running and jogging. Walking is a great exercise, and all you really need is a pair of walking shoes that fit well. You can get earphones and enjoy tape-recorded music while you walk, you can walk with a friend, or you can walk alone. If you live in a climate where it is sometimes too cold or rainy, and you want to walk, consider a shopping mall. A mall is a good place to walk, and many malls have organized walking clubs.

8. Be Realistic

We live in a very goal-oriented society. We set goals all the time; we're going to lose weight in two months, stop smoking in three, and transform ourselves into slim young lovelies in four. The goals are unrealistic, and invariably we fall short, become discouraged, and give up. Since no one knows you better than yourself, you should set realistic goals for yourself. Some examples might be:

- My goal is to be able to walk to the post office without huffing and puffing.
- My goal is to be able to exercise holding five-pound weights effortlessly.

- My goal is to keep up with my grandson when we go for a hike.

9. Underdo. Don't Overdo.

By far the biggest mistake people make when they begin exercising is to overdo it. You sign up for a bunch of exercise classes, or you decide to swim five days a week, or walk everywhere instead of taking the car. What happens? You exhaust yourself, become waterlogged, or get drenched in the rain. Before you know it, you're back on the couch again. So if you're busy, instead of trying to squeeze in an exercise class three times a week, find one that meets twice a week. You'll be more apt to stick with it, and that's what counts in the long run.

10. Viva Variety (Again)

Just as you try new foods, try different activities. Drop the ones you don't like, keep the ones you do, and try some different ones. It's a benefit that different types of activities use different parts of your body. Professional athletes call this cross-training. For example, a runner training for a marathon might run five days and then take a leisurely bike ride on the sixth day.

11. Always Have a Backup Plan

It is important to be able to switch to another activity if the need arises—if your exercise class has a break, your walking companion gets sick, or you mildly twist your ankle. In each of these cases, if you've planned ahead, you can switch to swimming, or some other activity, without skipping a beat.

12. Lower Your Standards

Often people new to athletic activities tend to compare themselves to the pros and become discouraged. We should compare ourselves only to ourselves, but we usually have unrealistic expectations of ourselves as well. So relax your standards! If your prowess at tennis consists mainly of running around the court chasing balls, but you enjoy it, that's fine. On the other hand, if feeling perennially klutzy is making you uncomfortable, consider finding an activity to which you are better suited, or take a few lessons. But remember, you don't have to be perfect!

Remember, increase your activity level gradually. If you're doing a mile on a treadmill, don't add another mile; start with adding on a quarter of a mile for, say, a week, then continue for a few weeks at one and a quarter miles, then add another quarter mile, and so on. If you stop exercising, when you resume, cut back significantly on your activities. It is sad but true that it does not take long at all for your body to begin getting out of condition again. So if you have to stop for a while, if you're ill, or even after a vacation, you'll have to start out slowly again.

Also, give yourself permission to slip (occasionally). Far too often we decide we are going to exercise for a given period of time. Then we go on vacation, get sick, or just bored, and miss a time or two. "That's it," we say to ourselves. "It's no use! Back to the couch!" Well, even if that happens, you can't stay on the couch forever. At some point, pick yourself up and go back to the health club or try another type of activity. The most difficult part of going back to a health club is returning for the first time. But almost everyone has been through a similar experience, and before you know it, you'll be back on track!

Beat Your Risk: *Exercise safely. If you walk or exercise outdoors, pick a safe area. Go with a friend and steer clear of high-crime areas. If you are choosing a health club, particularly if you are going to use it at night, make certain the parking lot is well lit and located in an area where you feel safe.*

THE BOTTOM LINE

There really is a fountain of youth, and that's exercise. Getting active is not easy—it takes time and work. But once you get into the habit, it can be a lot of fun. And it pays off big time in helping you to beat your risk.

CHAPTER 18

STEP 4: CONSIDER HORMONE REPLACEMENT THERAPY

ONE-THIRD OF AMERICA'S FEMALE POPULATION has now reached, or passed, menopause. Undoubtedly, many millions of these women are asking themselves "Should I, or shouldn't I take hormones?" It is a very real dilemma.

Your risk of heart disease, osteoporosis, and stroke—all major killers of women—mounts as you age. Hormone replacement therapy can play a role in reducing these threats. On the other hand, as your age climbs, your risk of breast cancer also mounts, and hormones may increase that risk. Therefore, this question has launched a vociferous debate—in thousands and thousands of pages of books and magazine articles as well as Internet newsgroups and websites devoted to menopause.

To make this all the more difficult, this is a question upon which experts disagree. For example, two of the most influential female doctors in the field of women's health today hold widely divergent views. Bernadine Healy, M.D., former director of the National Institutes of Health, writes, "When I hit menopause, I will begin HRT without a blink." Dr. Susan Love disagrees. When you pass menopause, she says, "you're not supposed to have hormones. You're not replacing something that's missing; it's not supposed to be there."

It's not surprising these experts clash; cardiologist Healy dearly wants to reduce heart disease in women, while breast surgeon Love is desperately concerned about adding to breast cancer's deadly toll.

Indeed, this is a difficult question without a crystal-clear answer. To make an informed decision, you need to consider the following facts.

WHAT IS MENOPAUSE?

Menopause is the time when your reproductive life ends. Although the average age is 51, menopause usually occurs between ages 41 and 55; a small percentage of women experience it before 40. The surgical removal of the ovaries can cause premature menopause; chemotherapy or radiation can do so as well.

The onset of menopause begins gradually with a period of subtle hormonal changes called the *climacteric*. This phase ends when estrogen levels fall so low that a woman experiences her final menstrual period.

The biological changes that occur during menopause are primarily due to the decline in the production of estrogen, the so-called female sex hormone. Once estrogen was thought to affect primarily a woman's reproductive system, but it is now becoming clear that estrogen may affect almost every other organ of the body as well, including the brain, breasts, heart, uterus, urinary tract, and bones.

You may have the impression that your estrogen production ceases, but that's not necessarily the case. Although the levels of estrogen and progesterone decline, causing your period to eventually stop, your adrenal glands still manufacture a hormonal substance known as *androstenedion*, which can be converted in the fat cells to a hormone that acts like estrogen. How long this continues varies among women, but it may be why some women experience less severe menopause symptoms than others. This hormonal production also may confer some of the physiological benefits of estrogen even after menopause. This is why striving to lose every ounce of excess weight may not be the best of health goals after all.

TYPES OF HORMONE REPLACEMENT THERAPY

Thanks to a proliferation in menopausal products, there are now several different types of hormone replacement therapy, and more are in the pipeline. Here's a rundown on four of the major classifications.

Estrogen replacement therapy (ERT) is the practice of giving pure, or unopposed, estrogen, the first type of hormonal replacement that came into use.

Hormone replacement therapy (HRT) is the combination of estrogen and progestin that is given to the vast majority of women who take hormones today. There are several such combination preparations on the market.

Selective estrogen receptor modulators (SERMs), known also as designer hormones, are therapies designed to prevent cardiovascular heart disease and osteoporosis but hopefully prevent breast and uterine cancer.

Plant-based estrogens—made from plants instead of from animal hormones—are another alternative. For instance, Estratab is a low-dose estrogen synthesized from soy and yams, which helps prevent bone loss, although not as much as higher doses of ERT or HRT or Fosamax do.

These are only some examples; the types of menopausal treatments are constantly expanding and changing. If you decide to use HRT, you need to discuss with your doctor the right product and formulation for you. The purpose of this chapter is to provide you with an understanding of the general use of hormones within the context of preventing disease.

SHORT-TERM HORMONE USE

"I'm exhausted. I've been having hot flashes so often that they wake me up. But I don't want to go on hormones because I'm afraid I'll get breast cancer," says 54-year-old Julie. She speaks in a tired voice; she is worn out by nights of tossing and turning, because her sleep is interrupted by the menopausal night sweats that awaken her.

Unfortunately, Julie's fears may be depriving her of relief. The controversy she referring to is not about short-term use of hormones. It's generally been found that taking them for up to five years and then tapering off is safe. You should taper off over a period of four to six months, though, or those hot flashes and other symptoms will return.

THE GREAT HORMONE DEBATE

The great hormone debate refers not to the short-term use of hormones but to their indefinite use by healthy women to prevent disease. To put this debate into perspective, you need to go back about 25 years. The idea of supplementing an aging woman's diminishing supply of estrogen isn't new. Synthetic hormones were developed in the early 1920s, but their popularity skyrocketed in the mid-1960s and early '70s, thanks to Robert A. Wilson, a gynecologist who promoted their use in his 1968 book *Feminine Forever*. But his claims were tarnished after the use of pure, unopposed estrogen (ERT) was found to increase a woman's risk of uterine cancer, known also as endometrial cancer. This was not considered an acceptable trade-off for hormone use.

Not long afterward, scientists discovered that this increased risk could be avoided if progestin, a synthetic form of progesterone, the other hormone produced during a woman's menstrual cycle, was administered too. Using a combination of estrogen and progestin, known as HRT, came into practice, with pure estrogen reserved only for women whose uteruses had been removed. Although HRT is believed to reduce uterine cancer, it doesn't eliminate the risk of breast cancer, which, for many women, is a good enough reason to refuse it. The hunt was on for a drug that would be the best of both worlds and deliver the benefits of HRT without the risk. Such a product was believed to have been discovered when the SERMs, a new class of drugs, came onto the market in the late 1990s.

These hormones take advantage of recent discoveries about the workings of estrogen. Although not fully understood, estrogen is known to produce its effect indirectly by stimulating the production of proteins that encourage cell growth and proliferation. In doing this, estrogen locks into a receptor molecule in the nucleus of the cell. In turn, the cell's receptor sends a signal that turns on the gene responsible for making a growth protein, giving estrogen its effect. These receptors are not exclusive; they can also pair up with other molecules that bear a resemblance to estrogen. When they do, they don't send the signal for protein production, and they become, in effect, estrogen blockers.

Scientists have been able to take advantage of this knowledge to create SERMs, which can be directed to bind to some estrogen receptors but block others. The first SERM was tamoxifen (Nolvadex), which was developed as a breast cancer treatment because it blocks estrogen receptors in breast cancer cells. The second, raloxifen (Evista) was approved by the FDA in 1996 as a form of hormone replacement therapy. The first of the so-called "designer" hormones, raloxifen stimulates estrogen receptors in the bones and liver, increasing bone mass and reducing LDL (bad) cholesterol, but blocks estrogen receptors in the breast and the uterus, so cancer risk is not increased at these sites. Indeed, raloxifen is being researched as a potential breast cancer preventative.

Researchers have long sought to find hormones that would produce cardiovascular and bone-saving benefits while not increasing cancer risks, and SERMs may prove to be this boon. But there are some concerns.

First, raloxifen was approved following clinical trials in which more than 12,800 women took the drug for over two and a half years. Some researchers worry that this wasn't a large enough group or a long enough trial period to rule out any possible increased cancer risks. After all, tamoxifen was hailed as a breast cancer wonder drug but later was found also to increase the risk of uterine cancer. There is also concern about other potential cancer risks down the road. For instance, raloxifen causes ovarian tumors in rats and mice, and Samuel S. Epstein, M.D., professor of environmental medicine at the University of Illinois School of Public Health, worries that this could occur in women as well. Eli Lilly and Company, which manufacturers the drug, takes issue with this contention, pointing out that the FDA has reviewed all the data, including animal trials, and judged the drug to be safe. Only time will tell if SERMs can deliver all that is promised.

A major randomized study, the Women's Health Initiative (WHI), currently is under way. This is not an observational study; it will compare groups of women taking the drugs with those on placebos. The study is designed to ferret out what the true benefits and risks of hormone replacement therapy are. However, as more and more menopause drugs are added to the roster, including formulations not included in the studies, the choices may become more complex.

Here is a rundown on what is currently known about the benefits, and the risks, of hormone replacement therapy.

THE BENEFITS OF HORMONE REPLACEMENT THERAPY

Heart Disease

Currently, the FDA approves the use of HRT for the prevention of osteoporosis, not heart disease. However, a great deal of the enthusiasm for HRT stems from the numerous studies that find that its use is associated with an estimated 30 to 50 percent decrease in the risk of heart disease in observational trials. The potential reduction represents an enormous number of women when you consider that more than 250,000 American women die of heart disease each year.

Furthermore, both ERT and HRT have been found to have multiple beneficial effects on the heart. First, information from laboratory studies as well as controlled trials indicates that HRT increases the HDL (good) cholesterol and lowers LDL (bad) cholesterol. In addition, HRT raises levels of substances that prevent blood clots in coronary arteries, and estrogen keeps the blood vessels more supple—both factors that reduce the risk of heart attack.

In addition, these benefits have repeatedly been shown to benefit women who have known risk factors for heart disease even more than women who do not. For instance, the Nurse's Health Study found that users of HRT who had one or more risk factors for heart disease experienced a 50 percent reduction in their death rate, compared to an 11 percent reduction in HRT users without risk factors, according to a study published in 1997 in the *New England Journal of Medicine*.

However, even enthusiastic supporters of HRT acknowledge that the largest benefits have come from observational studies, such as the Nurses' Health Study, and there are factors that might skew these results. For instance, women who regularly take HRT are more likely to have healthier profiles; they usually are thinner, exercise regularly, see their doctors more often, and so on, which may translate to a lower risk to begin with. In addition, a "healthy survivor" factor may exist, because women often stop taking HRT if they become acutely or seriously ill, thus creating a healthy survivor population of current users. Finally, the majority of studies have looked at women taking only ERT, which may have the strongest protective benefit, but it is now known that the majority of women must take HRT to protect themselves from uterine cancer.

However, even if the large reductions shown in these observational studies do not hold up, it is becoming more and more apparent that hormone use provides at least some benefit to the heart. After all, not all of the studies have been observational; the Postmenopausal Estrogen/Progestin(s) Intervention trial, known as the PEPI study, found that hormones, no matter which regimen, decreased heart disease risk, although not as much as was shown in the observational studies. This randomized study involved 875 healthy postmenopausal women who were placed on four different hormonal regimens. The results found that all the women taking hormones accrued a 20 percent reduction in LDL (bad) cholesterol and that their HDL (good) cholesterol was increased as well. Although the women who volunteered for the PEPI study presumably were more health-conscious than average, those taking placebos instead of hormones did not have as good results. "When it comes to HRT, mind over matter apparently is not good enough," commented Dr. Bernadine Healy, writing in a 1995 editorial published along with the study in the *Journal of the American Medical Association*.

Yet not all the studies have turned out as expected. The Heart and Estrogen/progestin Replacement Study (HERS) was designed to measure the effect of replacement hormones on women who already had heart disease. The study, conducted on 2,763 heart patients, tested whether taking various hormone regimens would cut the number of subsequent heart attacks these women suffered. To the surprise of the researchers, the study, published in 1998 in the *Journal of the American Medical Association*, found no significant difference between the two groups. There was a trend, as the study was winding down, for the women taking hormones to suffer fewer heart attacks, so the possibility exists that such drug use may be beneficial over the long run. But the sobering results of this study also demonstrate that the understanding of the impact of hormones on heart disease in women remains incomplete.

Osteoporosis

Because of the powerful benefit of HRT for the bones, many experts advocate its wider use, including Dr. Robert Lindsay at Columbia University. In his book *Osteoporosis*, Dr. Lindsay notes that studies have shown that women who took postmenopausal estrogen for six years or longer decreased their general risk of fracture by 50 to 60 percent. In fact, he believes hormone therapy could prevent a whopping 80 percent of spinal compression fractures and 50 percent of hip fractures.

Lila Wallis, M.D., at Cornell University Medical College, who is also the founding president of the National Council on Women's Health, takes a conservative approach. For instance, she notes that women at low risk for osteoporosis don't necessarily need hormones or any other type of osteoporosis preventative medication at all. For all women, especially those at high risk of osteoporosis, Dr. Wallis recommends lifestyle changes, mainly bone-strengthening exercises and making sure your vitamin D intake is adequate. If that is not enough, hormone replacement therapy or the nonhormonal medication Fosamax may be in order. For women at high risk of both osteoporosis and heart disease, hormone replacement therapy may help, she says.

Estrogen is also considered an important form of therapy because it can be started right at menopause, or even later, and still provide bone-maintaining benefits, notes Dr. Karl Insogna at the Yale Bone Center. "The important point is that even ten years after menopause it's not too late, because older women respond almost as well as younger women to estrogen. Of course, they can't rebuild all the bone they've lost, but they can still get a very good increase in bone mass."

Once estrogen is stopped, though, bone density begins to decline again, according to a 1993 study in the *New England Journal of Medicine*. This has led to the consideration of various options on when to start hormone replacement therapy, note Drs. Bruce Ettinger and Deborah Grady, in an editorial accompanying the study. They outline the following options:

- Start estrogen therapy at the time of menopause and never stop; this strategy would provide the most benefit and reduce fracture risk by an estimated two-thirds.
- Start estrogen treatment many years after menopause, when the risk of fracture is greatest, and continue it indefinitely. The drawback is that some preventable fractures might already have occurred.
- Start estrogen after an osteoporosis-induced fracture in hopes of reducing future fractures. Here, of course, some fractures would also have occurred.

These options can be weighed by a woman who is balancing the bone- and heart-saving benefits of hormone replacement therapy with the potential added breast cancer risk. In any case, the authors note, women should realize that "osteoporosis is unlikely to be prevented by taking estrogen for just a decade or so after menopause."

Estratab, the estrogen synthesized from soy and yams that was approved in 1998 for the prevention of osteoporosis, strengthens bones and improves cholesterol levels, but like estrogen, it carries an increased breast cancer risk and must be taken with progestin to lower the risk of uterine cancer. The SERM raloxifen is also approved for use as an osteoporosis preventative. It does strengthen bone, although to a lesser degree than estrogen, but hopefully does not carry an increased cancer risk.

Stroke

When they were first marketed, oral contraceptives containing large doses of estrogen were found to cause stroke. But formulas have changed, and now hormone replacement therapy is being considered a possible stroke preventative after menopause.

A Swedish study published in 1993 in the *Archives of Internal Medicine* examined the medical records of 23,088 women who took hormones during the late 1970s and found that, overall, less women than expected suffered strokes. The strongest reduction occurred in women who were recent users of hormones and began taking them at, or shortly after, menopause.

The study showed a risk reduction for those on both ERT and HRT. This is important, because it was feared that adding progestin might blunt the benefit. Earlier, a 1988 study in the *British Medical Journal* found that estrogen cut the risk of stroke by over 50 percent in 8,882 women.

The issue is by no means as clear-cut as in the case of heart disease. Not many studies have been done, and some find no risk reduction. Researchers don't know the mechanism by which hormones lower stroke risk, although the women in the Swedish study had slightly lower blood pressure, had less atherosclerosis (hardening of the arteries), and were at less risk for diabetes—all factors that could influence stroke risk. In addition, these are observational studies, as were those done for heart disease, so the women taking hormones may have had healthier lifestyles to begin with, skewing the results.

In animal studies, hormones apparently have a beneficial effect. A 1998 study published in *Stroke* found that the brain tissue of rats treated with estrogen and then made to suffer strokes sustained about half the brain damage of the control group. Will these findings hold up in humans? Studies are under way, including a major one at Yale Medical School in which 652 women who have suffered stroke, or are at high risk for stroke, will be evaluated. The study is not yet completed.

To sum up, currently it appears that hormone replacement therapy may provide some stroke protection, but this finding is not yet conclusive, and even if it does hold up, the protection will probably be less dramatic than that afforded for heart disease.

Colon Cancer

Although hormone replacement therapy is being studied the most for reducing heart disease, osteoporosis, and stroke, it may help reduce colon cancer as well. Researchers have suspected that hormones may influence the development of colon cancer since 1969, when it was reported that nuns suffered from a higher rate of colon cancer. It was presumed that this occurred because they did not undergo the hormonal changes that occur with pregnancy. Researchers pursuing this link got conflicting results, but a pair of studies published in 1995 in the *Journal of the National Cancer Institute* show that there may indeed be a protective effect.

The first study, published in April, found that women taking estrogen had a significantly reduced risk of dying from this potential killer. This large observational study, reviewing data from almost a half million postmenopausal women, found that the longer a woman took estrogen, the less likely she was to die of colon cancer.

This study is consistent with previous research, but there is some uncertainty over whether this benefit should be ascribed to the hormones. Because women taking hormones see their doctors more frequently, their cancers may have been diagnosed earlier, saving their lives. Furthermore, women who take hormones are usually more health conscious and live a healthier lifestyle, so another factor could be involved.

This study focused only on women who took ERT. The second study, published a few months later, reported on those who took HRT. This study compared 694 female colon cancer patients with other women and also found that those on hormones were at sharply reduced risk.

If hormones are bestowing the benefit, researchers are unsure why. However, they speculate that these hormones may help reduce the concentration of bile acids in the stomach, which may promote tumors.

THE RISKS OF HORMONE REPLACEMENT THERAPY

Breast Cancer

For many women, the demonstrated bone-strengthening properties of HRT, the promises of a healthier heart, and other potential health benefits pale if it increases the risk of breast cancer. Using HRT can increase this risk over a woman's lifetime from an estimated 10 percent to 13-17 percent. Some critics contend that this is an underestimate; a woman's relative risk may be as high as 35 percent.

Fears about a possible link between estrogen replacement therapy and breast cancer were sparked by a 1989 Swedish study that found a significant increase in the risk of breast cancer for 23,244 women taking estrogen. Since then numerous studies have been done, with some finding significantly increased risk, others none at all, and many others landing in between.

For instance, a pair of studies published a month apart in 1995 found very different results. The first study, published in the *New England Journal of Medicine*, was based on the Nurses' Health Study, using observational data from over 121,000 participants. The most added risk was found for women over the age of 55 who had been on HRT for over five years. The second study, reported a month later in the *Journal of the American Medical Association*, compared 537 breast cancer patients with 492 randomly selected healthy women and found no correlation between taking HRT and getting breast cancer. However, it should be noted that this was a much smaller study.

Almost everyone, including those who tout HRT for osteoporosis and heart disease, acknowledges that using hormones for over five years does increase the risk of breast cancer. But experts vary. Some find such risk figures tolerable, given the vast numbers of women who could be saved from heart attacks. Graham Colditz, M.D., associate professor of medicine at Harvard Medical School, disagrees. He contends that many observational studies have underestimated the risk of breast cancer posed by HRT. His analysis of all studies, including international research, published in 1998 in the *Journal of the National Cancer Institute,* found a 35 percent increase in relative risk for current users of HRT who had been on it for over five years.

He notes that there is a contention that "HRT is great to reduce the risk of heart disease, therefore everyone should use it." He points out that women can do many things to reduce their risk of heart disease, such as making changes in diet and exercise, "but there aren't many things that a woman can do to reduce her risk of breast cancer."

Hopefully, the hormones in the SERMs class will not raise breast cancer risk. But, as noted earlier, these drugs have not been around that long, and their true benefits, as well as their risks, are not yet definitively known.

Ovarian Cancer

As noted in chapter 9, there is concern that using hormones may raise the risk of ovarian cancer, but definitive proof is lacking. Researchers speculate that the use of postmenopausal estrogen could promote the overgrowth of cells in the ovary, which may then result in cancer. This theory is similar to HRT's link to breast cancer, but with ovarian cancer, the tie is much more tenuous because research findings are contradictory.

For instance, a 1995 study published in the *American Journal of Epidemiology* found that women who took replacement estrogen for at least six years had a 40 percent higher risk of dying from ovarian cancer. Furthermore, those who used the hormone for 11 years had an increased risk of 70 percent.

This large-scale American Cancer Society study reviewed data from 676,526 women. However, the study's authors caution that their research has limitations. First, many of the women in the study took higher doses of estrogen than are currently used today. Second, the study did not look at women who take a combination of estrogen and progesterone, the most common regimen in use today. Therefore, they noted, more research is needed among these groups.

Furthermore, not all studies have found such a risk. For instance, an analysis of 12 studies published in 1992 in the same journal found no clear association with estrogen and ovarian cancer. The only exception was one study that found increased risk among a small number of women who had also used diethylstilbestrol (DES).

Uterine (Endometrial) Cancer

As noted earlier, it was discovered some 20 years ago that unopposed estrogen increased a woman's risk of uterine, or endometrial, cancer. This was confirmed as part of the PEPI trial, which noted in 1996 that the women in the group who were given ERT were far more likely to develop some type of endometrial hyperplasia—the changes in the lining of the cells that can lead to uterine cancer.

Beat Your Risk: *If you still have your uterus, you should not take estrogen without a progestin. It may be tempting to, because it is progestin that often causes unwelcome side effects of HRT, such as breast tenderness. But the progestin is necessary to lower the risk of uterine cancer.*

Blood Clots

Although most of the discussion about the risks of HRT center on breast cancer, studies have found there also is a two- to fourfold increase in the risk of venous thromboembolism, or blood clots that can form in the veins of the legs and travel to the lungs. This increased risk appears to be greatest at the start of therapy and applies to women who weigh more. This means it is not a major risk factor for most women.

YOUR DECISION ABOUT HRT

So many books, magazines, and discussions address the question of hormone replacement therapy, you may feel compelled to make a decision. You don't necessarily have to. If you are at low, or even average, risk for osteoporosis and heart disease, this decision may not even be an issue for you.

"Part of the advertising and promotion of hormones is that every woman has this burning decision to make. But if a woman feels well during menopause, if she has no reason to fear early osteoporosis or heart disease, she may have no decision to make," says Barbara Seaman, a founder of the women's health movement and author of many books, including the reissued *Doctor's Case Against the Pill*.

On the other hand, if you are at high risk for osteoporosis or heart disease, taking hormones after menopause may be wise. How do you know this is the right decision for you? There really isn't a definite yes or no answer at this point. The best thing to do, the experts advise, is to weigh your personal risk factors, along with the other facts.

To Make Your Long-Term Decision about HRT

- Weigh your personal risk-benefit profile. If you've been answering this book's quizzes and charting your family medical tree, you have a far greater idea of that than most. By using the rest of the information in this chapter, you can then evaluate how hormones may increase or reduce that risk.

- Make your decision on a short-term basis and be prepared to reevaluate it. Many women feel that they need to make a decision about hormones *now* that they will stick with for their whole lives. This is usually not the case. You can reevaluate your decision based on new medical findings or changes in your risk factors, or simply because you wish to, anytime you want.

- If you do opt for HRT, make sure you're on the smallest dose that is supposed to give the preventative effects you are seeking.

- If you opt for HRT, monitor your breast cancer risk by doing regular self-exams, having annual breast exams by a health professional, and having annual mammograms.

- Don't neglect other healthy lifestyle changes. Studies indicate that HRT may give you an edge in warding off some diseases, but it's not a magic bullet that erases the effects of an unhealthy lifestyle. Research has found, for instance, that combining HRT with exercise provides the most protection against osteoporosis and heart disease.

Which Women Should *Not* Take HRT

Hormones are usually not indicated for certain groups of women. These are women with:

- Current breast cancer
- Current endometrial cancer
- Current ovarian cancer
- Active liver disease
- Active thrombophlebitis or thromboembolism (these are conditions associated with blood clots)

Hormones are generally not advised for women who have suffered strokes or transient ischemic attacks (TIA), although research in this area is currently under way. If you have vaginal bleeding from an unknown cause, it must be diagnosed before going on hormones (actually, this is a symptom that should be checked out in any case).

Discuss Hormone Therapy with Your Doctor If You Have:

- Large uterine fibroids
- Endometriosis
- High blood pressure (that is aggravated by estrogen)

Other Considerations

- *Migraine.* Women who suffer so-called menstrual migraines may find that hormones can worsen these symptoms. However, adjusting the levels of estrogen and progestin can help this problem.
- *Gallbladder Disease.* Some studies indicate that estrogen may increase the risk of gallstones.

If You're a Cancer Survivor

Women who have had certain types of cancer, particularly breast cancer, have long been told they should not take postmenopausal hormones. However, chemotherapy and radiation often propels these women into early menopause, which can be accompanied by severe menopausal symptoms. Studies are currently under way to learn if these women can safely take HRT, so discuss this with your doctor.

THE BOTTOM LINE

Most experts agree that the only way to make a decision about HRT, given the current climate of uncertainty, is to weigh your individual risk factors.

RESOURCES

Books

Breast Cancer

Baron-Faust, Rita. *Breast Cancer: What Every Woman Should Know.* New York: Hearst Books, 1995.

Love, Susan M., M.D., with Karen Lindsey. *Dr. Susan Love's Breast Cancer Book.* 2nd ed. Reading, Mass.: Addison-Wesley, 1995.

Swirsky, Joan, and Barbara Balaban. *The Breast Cancer Handbook.* New York: HarperCollins, 1994.

Cancer

McGinn, Kerry A., R.N., and Pamela J. Haycock, R.N. *Women's Cancers: How to Prevent Them, How to Treat Them, How to Beat Them.* Alameda, Calif.: Hunter House, 1998.

Compulsive Eating

Bruno, Barbara Altman. *Worth Your Weight: What You Can Do about a Weight Problem.* Bethel, Conn.: Rutledge, 1996.

Orbach, Susie. *Fat Is a Feminist Issue: The Anti-Diet Guide for Women.* New York: Berkley, 1994.

Diet and Nutrition

Brody, Jane. *Jane Brody's Nutrition Book: A Lifetime Guide to Good Eating and Better Health and Weight Control.* New York, Bantam, 1988.

Nelson, Miriam E., Ph.D., with Sarah Wernick, Ph.D. *Strong Women Stay Slim.* New York: Bantam, 1998.

Cookbooks

American Heart Association Quick and Easy Cookbook. New York: Times Books, 1995.

Jenkins, Nancy Harmon. *The Mediterranean Diet Cookbook: A Delicious Alternative for Lifelong Health.* New York: Bantam, 1994.

Robertson, Robin. *The Soy Gourmet.* New York: Plume, 1998.

Winter, Ruth, M.S. *Super Soy: The Miracle Bean.* New York: Crown, 1996.

Exercise

Price, Joan, M.A. *Joan Price Says, Yes, You Can Get in Shape! Make Exercise a Treat, Not a Treatment.* Pacifica, Calif.: Pacifica Press, 1996.

Nelson, Miriam E., Ph.D., with Sarah Wernick, Ph.D. *Strong Women Stay Young.* New York: Bantam, 1997.

General Medicine

The Merck Manual of Medical Information Home Edition. West Point, Pa.: Merck, 1997.

Genetics and Genealogy (Family History)

Krause, Carol. *How Healthy Is Your Family Tree: A Complete Guide to Tracing Your Family's Medical and Behavioral History.* New York: Simon and Schuster, 1995.

Milunsky, Aubrey, M.D. *Heredity and Your Family's Health.* Baltimore: Johns Hopkins Univ. Press, 1992.

"Where to Write for Vital Records" (free pamphlet). Superintendent of Documents, U.S. Government Printing Office, Washington, D.C., 20402.

Heart Disease

Pashkow, Fredric J., and Charlotte Libov. *Fifty Essential Things to Do When the Doctor Says It's Heart Disease*. New York: Plume, 1995.

Menopause and Hormone Replacement Therapy

Love, Susan M., M.D., with Karen Lindsey. *Dr. Susan Love's Hormone Book*. New York: Random House, 1997.

Nachtigall, Lila, M.D., and Joan Rattner Heilman. *Estrogen: The Facts Can Change Your Life*. New York: HarperCollins, 1995.

Notelovitz, Morris, M.D., and Diana Tonnessen. *Menopause and Midlife Health*. New York: St. Martin's Press, 1993.

Sachs, Judith. *What Women Should Know about Menopause*. New York, Dell, 1991.

Utian, Wulf H., and Ruth S. Jacobowitz. *Managing Your Menopause*. New York: Prenctice Hall Press, 1990.

Medical Resources

Linden, Tom, M.D., and Michelle L. Kienholz. *Dr. Tom Linden's Guide to Online Medicine*. New York: McGraw-Hill, 1995. You can sample the book by checking out Dr. Linden's Web page at http://www.mcgraw-hill.com; click on "Professional and Reference Groups."

Osteoporosis

Notelovitz, Morris, M.D., Ph.D. *Stand Tall: Every Woman's Guide to Preventing and Treating Osteoporosis*. Gainesville, Fl.: Triad, 1998.

Radon

For information on how to test for and remove radon from your home, contact the Environmental Protection Agency, Information Access Branch, Public Information Center at 202-260-2080.

Stress Reduction

Davis, M., E.R. Eshelman, and M. McKay. *The Relaxation and Stress Reduction Workbook*. 3rd ed. Oakland, Calif.: New Harbinger, 1988.

Women's Health

Boston Women's Health Collective. *The New Our Bodies, Ourselves*. New York: Simon and Schuster, 1992.

Healy, Bernadine, M.D. *A New Prescription for Women's Health: Getting the Best Medical Care in a Man's World*. New York: Viking, 1995.

Hoffman, Eileen, M.D. *Our Health, Our Lives: A Revolutionary Approach to Total Health Care for Women*. New York: Pocket, 1995.

Laurence, Leslie, and Beth Weinhouse. *Outrageous Practices: The Alarming Truth about How Medicine Mistreats Women*. New York: Fawcett, 1994.

Newsletters

Harvard Women's Health Watch
P.O. Box 420234
Palm Coast, FL 32142-0234

Heart Advisor
P.O. Box 420235
Palm Coast, FL 32142-0235
800-829-2506

Ovarian Plus International Newsletter
P.O. Box 498
Paauilo, HI 96776-0498

Women's Health Hot Line
http://www.libov.com
Free Internet newsletter offering health news for women, founded and edited by Charlotte Libov.

Organizations and Support Groups

Adoption
Adoption Liberty Movement Association
P.O. Box 154
Washington Bridge Station
New York, NY 10033

Breast Cancer

Massachusetts Breast Cancer Coalition
Two Boylston Street
Boston, MA 02116
1-800-649-2222; 617-423-6222

Mothers Supporting Daughters with Breast Cancer
c/o Charmayne Dierker
21710 Bayshore Road
Chestertown, MD 21650
410-778-1982

National Alliance of Breast Cancer Organizations
9 East 37th Street, 10th Floor
New York, NY 10016
212-889-4923

National Coalition for Breast Cancer Survivorship
1010 Wayne Avenue, 5th Floor
Silver Spring, MD 20910
301-650-8868

Women of Color Breast Cancer Survivors Project
8610 Sepulveda Boulevard, Suite 200
Los Angeles, CA 90045
310–216–3200

Cancer

American Cancer Society
1599 Clifton Road, N.E.
Atlanta, GA 30329-4251
1-800-ACS-2345; 404-320-3333
http://www.cancer.org
Also offers the "Fresh Start" Smoking Cessation program.

National Cancer Institute
Cancer Information Service
9000 Rockville Pike
Bethesda, MD 20892
1-800-4-CANCER; 301-496-5583

Consumer Education

For a free catalog listing of government publications which are free or very inexpensive and include health topics, write to the Consumer Education Center, P.O. Box 100, Pueblo, CO 81002.

DES

DES Action
1615 Broadway, Suite 510
Oakland, CA 94612
1-800-DES-9288

DES Cancer Network
Box 10185
Rochester, NY 14610
1-800-DES NET4

Diabetes

American Diabetes Association
1600 Duke Street
Alexandria, VA 11324
1-800-232-3472
http://www.diabetes.org

National Diabetes Information Clearinghouse
One Information Way
Bethesda, MD 20892-3560
301-654-3327

Exercise and Fitness

President's Council on Physical Fitness and Sports
701 Pennsylvania Avenue, Suite 250
Washington, DC 20004
202-272-3421

General Medicine

These organizations have information on a variety of health issues, and in particular their Internet sites generally also have worthwhile links.

The American Medical Association
515 North State Street
Chicago, IL 60610
312-464-5000
http://www.ama-assn.org

The Centers for Disease Control and Prevention
1600 Clifton Road, N.E.
Altanta, GA 30333
404-639-3311
http://www.cdc.gov

National Institutes of Health
9000 Rockville Pike
Bethesda, MD 20892
301-496-4000
http://www.nih.gov

U.S. Department of Health and Human Services
200 Independence Avenue, S.W.
Washington, DC 20201
202-619-0257
http://www.os.dhhs.gov

Genetic Diseases

Alliance of Genetic Support Groups
35 Wisconsin Circle, Suite 440
Chevy Chase, MD 20015
1-800-336-GENE; 301-652-5553
http://medhlp.netusa.net/www.agsg.htm

March of Dimes Birth Defects Foundation
National Office
1275 Mamaroneck Avenue
White Plains, NY 10605
914-428-7100

The Hereditary Center Institute
Creighton University School of Medicine
2500 California Plaza
Omaha, NE 68178
http://medicine.creighton.edu
402-280-1796

The National Society of Genetic Counselors
233 Canterbury Drive
Wallingford, PA 19086-6671

The NSGC will send a brochure, a list of certified genetic counselors who specialize in cancer counseling, and the names of nearby centers for genetic counseling. Prefers written request; no phone calls.

Heart Disease

American Heart Association
731 Greenville Avenue
Dallas, TX 75231
1-800-227-2345; 214-373-6300
www.amhrt.org

Coronary Club
9500 Euclid Avenue, A42
Cleveland, OH 44195
1-800-478-4255

National Heart, Lung and Blood Institute (NHLBI)
Information Center
P.O. Box 30105
Bethesda, MD 20824-0105
1-800-575-WELL; 301-251-1222

The NHLBI offers recorded messages and free information about controlling blood pressure, cholesterol levels, and other risk factors for heart disease.

Lesbian Health

National Gay and Lesbian Health Foundation
1638 R Street, N.W., Suite 2
Washington, DC 20009
202-939-7880

Lung Cancer

American Lung Association
1740 Broadway
New York, NY 10019
1-800-586-4872; 212-315-8700
http://www.lungusa.org
(Offers free smoking cessation material.)

Minority Health Issues

American Indian Health Care Association
245 E. 6th Street, Suite 499
St. Paul, MN 55101
612-294-0233

Asian American Health Forum
116 New Montgomery Street, Suite 531
San Francisco, CA 94105
415-541-0866

National Black Women's Health Project
1237 Ralph D. Abernathy Boulevard, S.W.
Atlanta, GA 30310
1-800-ASK-BWHP

National Coalition of Hispanic Health and Human Services
Organizations
1501 16th Street, N.W.
Washington, DC 20036-1401
203-387-5000

Office of Minority Health Resource Center
P.O. Box 37337
Washington, DC 20013-7337
800-444-6472

Nutrition

American Dietetic Association
216 West Jackson Boulevard
Chicago, IL 60606-6995
312-899-0040
312-899-1979 (fax)
www.eatright.org

Osteoporosis

National Osteoporosis Foundation
2100 M Street, N.W., Suite 602
Washington, DC 20011
202-223-2226; 1-800-223-9994
http://www.nof.org
Toll-free hot line on where to get a bone mass density test:
1-800-464-6700

Ovarian Cancer

Gilda Radner Familial Ovarian Cancer Registry
Roswell Park Cancer Institute
Elm and Carlton Streets
Buffalo, NY 14263
1-800-OVARIAN

Stroke

American Heart Association. See under "Heart Disease."

National Institute of Neurological Disorders and Stroke
9000 Rockville Pike, Building 31, Room 8A-06
Bethesda, MD 20992
1-800-852-9424

National Stroke Association
300 East Hampden Avenue, Suite 240
Englewood, CO 80110-2622
1-800-787-6537
http://www.stroke.org

Weight Issues

Largesse, the Network for Size Esteem
P.O. Box 9404
New Haven, CT 06534-0404
For women striving to accept their size.

Women's Health Issues

National Women's Health Network
514 10th Street, N.W., Suite 400
Washington, DC 20004
202-628-7814
Membership begins at $25. The NWHN publishes packets filled with articles about selected women's health topics that can be ordered for a nominal charge by both members and nonmembers.

The Older Women's League (OWL)
666 Eleventh Street, N.W., Suite 700
Washington, DC 20001
202-783-6686
A Washington D.C.–based organization that promotes older women's issues; publishes several free reports on women's health issues, including heart disease and osteoporosis.

Smoking—How to Quit

Books

Fisher, Edwin B., Jr., Ph.D., with Toni L. Goldfarb. *Seven Steps to a Smoke-Free Life*. New York: John Wiley, 1998.

Klesges, Robert C., PhD., and Margaret DeBon, M.S. *How Women Can Finally Stop Smoking*. Alameda, Calif.; Hunter House Publishers, 1994.

Pamphlets

Many free publications on the hazards of smoking and how to quit are available for free from the Centers for Disease Control and Prevention Office on Smoking and Health. To request one or more, write to the following address:

Office on Smoking and Health
Mail Stop K-50
4770 Buford Highway, N.E.
Altanta, GA 30341-3724
404-488-5705

The following is a sampling of the brochures and information available. The Centers for Disease Control also have several full-length reports on smoking from the surgeon general's office.

"Clearing the Air": Tips on smoking cessation from the National Cancer Institute.
"Good News for Smokers Fifty and Older": A fact sheet outlining the health benefits of quitting smoking.
"Out of the Ashes": Outlines various methods of quitting smoking.
"Pathways to Freedom": A smoking cessation program geared to African Americans.
"Reducing the Health Risks of Secondhand Smoke." A pamphlet from the American Lung Association and the Centers for Disease Control that describes ways to avoid secondhand smoke at home, at work, and in public places.

Also from the Centers for Disease Control, here's a list of agencies and nonprofit organizations that provide more information about smoking and health:

The Environmental Protection Agency offers publications and information on the adverse effects of environmental tobacco smoke and indoor air pollution.

Environmental Protection Agency
Indoor Air Quality Information Clearinghouse
P.O. Box 37133
Washington, DC 20013-7133

The National Cancer Institute supports research on tobacco control interventions, produces publications for health professionals and the public, and provides telephone counseling services for smoking cessation.

National Cancer Institute
Building 31, Room 10A24
9000 Rockville Pike
Bethesda, MD 20892
1-800-4-CANCER

The National Clearinghouse for Alcohol and Drug Information provides information about the health risks of using addictive drugs, including tobacco. Information is available in various forms, including videos, fact sheets, posters, and pamphlets.

Center for Substance Abuse Prevention
National Clearinghouse for Alcohol and Drug Information
P.O. Box 2345
Rockville, MD 20852
(301) 468-2600
1-800-Say-No-To

The National Heart, Lung, and Blood Institute develops smoking intervention resources for physicians and health care providers.

National Heart, Lung, and Blood Institute
P.O. Box 30105
Bethesda, MD 20824-0105
301-951-3260

The National Institute of Occupational Safety and Health provides information on secondhand smoke and other occupational safety and health concerns.

Centers for Disease Control and Prevention
National Institute for Occupational Safety and Health
4676 Columbia Parkway
Mailstop C-19
Cincinnati, OH 45226-1998
1-800-35-NIOSH

State and local health departments provide a variety of smoking and health information to the public. Check the government section of your phone book for current numbers and addresses.

Organizations

Action on Smoking and Health
2013 H Street, N.W.
Washington, DC 20006
202-659-4310

The Advocacy Institute works on efforts to counter the influence of the tobacco industry and provides strategic consulting and advocacy support on policy issues related to tobacco control.

The Advocacy Institute
Suite 600
1730 Rhode Island Avenue, N.W.
Washington, DC 20036-4505
202-659-8475

The American Association of Retired Persons maintains a resource list for health professionals and publishes a newsletter that addresses smoking cessation and health promotion.

American Association of Retired Persons
Elder Care Institute on Health Promotion and Aging
601 E Street, N.W.
Washington, DC 20049
202-434-2203

The American Cancer Society provides smoking education, prevention and cessation programs and distributes pamphlets, posters, and other materials on smoking. Refer to your phone book for the office in your area or contact the national office for further information; see the listing under "Cancer." ,

The American Heart Association promotes smoking intervention programs at schools, workplaces, and health care sites. Refer to your phone book for the chapter in your area or contact the national office for further information; see the listing under "Heart Disease."

The American Lung Association (ALA) conducts programs addressing smoking cessation, prevention, and the protection of nonsmokers' health and provides a variety of educational materials for the public and health professionals. Refer to your phone book for the ALA chapter in your area or contact the national office for further information; see the listing under "Lung Cancer."

The American Medical Association provides smoking intervention guides for physicians and health care providers; see the listing under "General Medicine."

Americans for Nonsmokers' Rights provides information to organizations and individuals to assist in passing ordinances, implementing workplace regulations, and developing smoking policies in the workplace.

Americans for Nonsmokers' Rights
2530 San Pablo Avenue, Suite J
Berkeley, CA 94702
510-841-3032

The Coalition on Smoking OR Health suports agencies in need of policy options and legislative assistance. Represents the American Cancer Society, American Heart Association, and American Lung Association.

Coalition on Smoking OR Health
1150 Connecticut Avenue, N.W., Suite 820
Washington, DC 20036
202-452-1184

The Group Against Smokers' Pollution (GASP) provides educational materials and information and referral services concerning the health hazards of secondhand smoke and the establishment of nonsmoking laws and policies.

Group Against Smokers' Pollution
P.O. Box 632
College Park, MD 20740
301-459-4791

The March of Dimes Birth Defects Foundation distributes health educational materials to the public, including materials about the effects of smoking during pregnancy; see the listing under "Genetic Diseases."

SmokeFree Educational Services, Inc., provides smoking and health educational materials for schools and workplaces in the form of booklets, posters, videos, and stickers.

SmokeFree Educational Services, Inc.
375 South End Avenue, Suite 32F
New York, NY 10280
212-912-0960

SELECTED BIBLIOGRAPHY

Books

Boston Women's Health Collective. *The New Our Bodies, Ourselves.* New York: Simon and Schuster, 1992.

DeGregorio, Michael W., and Valerie J. Wiebe. *Tamoxifin and Breast Cancer: What Everyone Should Know about the Treatment of Breast Cancer.* New Haven: Yale Univ. Press, 1994.

Kelly, Patricia T., Ph.D. *Understanding Breast Cancer Risk.* Philadelphia: Temple Univ. Press, 1991.

Lindsay, Robert, M.B.Ch.B, Ph.D., F.R.C.P. *Osteoporosis: A Guide to Diagnosis, Prevention and Treatment.* New York: Raven Press, 1992.

Love, Susan M., M.D., with Karen Lindsey. *Dr. Susan Love's Breast Book.* 2nd ed. Reading, Mass.: Addison-Wesley, 1995.

McGinn, Kerry A., R.N., and Pamela J. Haycock, R.N. *Women's Cancers: How to Prevent Them, How to Treat Them, How to Beat Them.* Alameda, Calif.: Hunter House, 1993.

Wallis, Lila A., M.D. *Modern Breast and Pelvic Examinations: A Handbook for Health Professionals.* New York: National Council on Women's Health, Inc., 1993.

Winawer, Sidney J., M.D., and Moshe Shike, M.D. *Cancer Free.* New York: Simon and Schuster, 1995.

Pamphlets and Publications

"A Different Perspective on Breast Cancer Risk Factors: Some Implications of the Non-Attributable Risk." American Cancer Society, 1983.

"A Status Report on Osteoporosis: The Challenge to Midlife and Older Women." Older Women's League, 1994.

"Breast Cancer Facts and Figures." American Cancer Society, 1997.

"Cancer Facts and Figures—1998." American Cancer Society, 1998.

"Cancer Facts and Figures for African Americans." American Cancer Society, 1996.

"Cancer of the Colon and Rectum: Research Report." National Cancer Institute, 1991.

Cancer of the Lung: Research Report." National Cancer Institute, 1993.

"DES Daughters." National Cancer Institute, National Institute of Child Health and Human Development, National Institutes of Health, 1995.

"Heart and Stroke Facts: 1997 Statistical Supplement." American Heart Association, 1996.

"Postmenopausal Hormone-Replacement Therapy." Harvard Health Publications Special Report, *Harvard Women's Health Watch*, 1996.

Ward, Darrell E. "Reporting on Cancer: A Guide for Journalists," Ohio State University Office of University Communications, 1994.

"Were You Born Between 1938 and 1971?" National Cancer Institute, National Institute of Child Health and Human Development, National Institutes of Health, 1995.

"Women and Smoking." *World Smoking and Health*, American Cancer Society, vol. 16, no. 2, 1991.

Consensus Statements

"Consensus Development Conference: Diagnosis, Prohylaxis and Treatment of Osteoporosis." *American Journal of Medicine*, vol. 94, June, 1993, pp. 646-50.

"Ovarian Cancer: Screening, Treatment, and Follow Up." *NIH Consensus Statement*, National Institutes of Health, vol. 12, no. 3, April 5-7, 1994.

"Sunlight, Ultraviolet Radiation and the Skin." *NIH Consensus Statement*, NIH, vol. 7, no. 8, May 8-10, 1989.

Articles

Airhihenbuwa, Collins, O., Shiriki Kumanyika, Tanya D. Agurs, and Agatha Lowe. "Perceptions and Beliefs about Exercise, Rest, and Health among African-Americans." *American Journal of Health Promotion*, vol. 9, no. 6, July/August 1995, pp. 426-429.

Alberts, Mark J., M.D., Lawrence M. Brass, M.D., April Perry, R.N., Debbie Webb, R.N., and Deborah V. Dawson, Ph.D. "Evaluation Time for Patients with In-Hospital Strokes." *Stroke*, vol. 24, no. 12, December 1993, pp. 1817-1821.

Al-Hani, Arfan J., M.D. "Women Take Heart: A Pioneering Study of Women's Health." Presented at the American Heart Association's 22nd Science Writers Forum, Santa Barbara, Calif., Jan. 15-18, 1995.

Alpha-Tocopherol, Beta Carotene Cancer Prevention Study Group. "The Effect of Vitamin E and Beta Carotene on the Incidence of Lung Cancer and Other Cancers in Male Smokers." *New England Journal of Medicine*, vol. 330, no. 15, April 14, 1994, pp. 1029-1035.

Anderson, James W., M.D., and Belinda M. Smith, M.S., R.D. "Fantastic Fiber." *Women's Health Digest*, vol. 1, no. 1, Winter 1995, pp. 24-27.

Anderson, James W., M.D., Bryan M. Johnstone, Ph.D., and Margaret E. Cook-Newell, M.S., R.D. "Meta-analysis of the Effects of Soy Protein on Serum Lipids." *New England Journal of Medicine*, vol. 333, no. 5, August 3, 1995, pp. 276-281.

Baines, Cornelia J., M.D., Marjan Vidmar, M.D., Gail McKeown-Cyssen, M.D., and Robert Tibshirani, Ph.D. "Impact of Menstrual Phase on False-Negative Mammograms in the Canadian National Breast Screening Study." *Cancer*, vol. 80, no. 4, August 15, 1997, pp. 720-724.

Baker, Trudy R., M.D., and M. Steven Piver, M.D. "Ovarian Cancer: The Genetic Link." *The Female Patient*, vol. 16, September 1991, pp. 87-92.

Barlow, Carolyn E., Harold W. Kohl, III, Larry W. Gibbons, and Steven

N. Blair. "Physical Fitness, Mortality and Obesity." *International Journal of Obesity*, supplement 4, 1995, pp. 541-544.

Barnes, Deborah E., M.P.H., and Lisa A. Bero, Ph.D. "Why Review Articles on the Health Effects of Passive Smoking Reach Different Conclusions." *Journal of the American Medical Association*, vol. 279, no. 19, May 20, 1998, pp. 1566-1570.

Beckett, William S., M.D., M.P.H. "Lung Cancer in Women: Selected Topics in Epidemiology and Prevention." *Journal of Women's Health*, vol. 4, no. 6, December 1995, pp. 637-643.

Berrino, Franco, Paolo Muti, Andrea Micheli, Gianfranco Bolelli, Vittorio Krogh, Raffalla Sciajno, Paola Pisani, Salvatore Panico, and Giorgio Secreto. "Serum Sex Hormone Levels after Menopause and Subsequent Breast Cancer." *Journal of the National Cancer Institute*, vol. 88, no. 5, March 6, 1996, pp. 291-296.

Bilimoria, Malcolm M., M.D., and Monica Morrow, M.D. "The Woman at Increased Risk for Breast Cancer: Evaluation and Management Strategies." *CA—A Cancer Journal for Clinicians*, vol. 45, no. 5, September/October 1995, pp. 263-278.

Black, Homer S., Ph.D., J. Alan Herd, M.D., Leonard H. Goldberg, M.D., John E. Wolf, Jr., M.D., John I. Thornby, Ph.D., Theodore Rosen, M.D., Suzanne Bruce, M.D., Jaime A. Tschen, M.D., John P. Foreyt, Ph.D., Lynne W. Scott, M.A., R.D., Suzanne Jaax, M.S., R.D., and Kelly Andrews, B.A. "Effect of a Low-Fat Diet on the Incidence of Actinic Keratosis." *New England Journal of Medicine*, vol. 330, no. 18, pp. 1273-1275.

Boyd, Jeff. "BRAC1: More than a Hereditary Breast Cancer Gene." *Nature Genetics*, vol. 9, April 1995, pp. 335-336.

Brass, Lawrence M., M.D., Jonathan L. Isaccsohn, M.D., Kathleen R. Merikangas, Ph.D., and C. Dennis Robinette, Ph.D. "A Study of Twins and Stroke." *Stroke*, vol. 23, no. 2, February 1992, pp. 221-223.

Brown, Harriet. "The Other Reward of Exercise." *Health*, July/August, 1994, pp. 34-36.

Browner, Warren S., M.D., M.P.H., Alice R. Pressman, M.S., Michael C. Nevitt, Ph.D., Jane A. Cauley, P.H., and Steven R. Cummings, M.D. "Association between Low Bone Density and Stroke in Elderly Women." *Stroke*, vol. 24, no. 7, July 1993, pp. 940-946.

Budoff, Matthew J., M.D., Demetrios Georgio, M.D., Alan Brody, M.D., Arthur S. Agatston, M.D., John Kennedy, M.D., Christopher

Wolfkiel, Ph.D., William Stanford, M.D., Paul Shields, M.D., Roger L. Lewis, M.D., Ph.D., Warren R. Janowitz, M.D., Stuart Rich, M.D., and Bruce H. Brundage, M.D. "Ultrafast Computed Tomography as a Diagnostic Modality in the Detection of Coronary Artery Disease." *Circulation*, vol. 93, no. 5, March 1, 1996, pp. 898-904.

Byers, Tim, M.D., M.P.H., Bernard Levin, M.D., David Rothenberger, M.D., Gerald D. Dodd, M.D., and Robert A. Smith, Ph.D. "American Cancer Society Guidelines for Screening and Surveillance for Early Detection of Colorectal Polyps and Cancer: Update 1997." *CA—A Cancer Journal for Clinicians*, vol. 47, no. 3, May/June 1997, pp. 154-160.

Calle, Eugenia E., Heidi L. Miracle-McMahill, Michael J. Thun, and Clark W. Heath, Jr. "Cigarette Smoking and Risk of Fatal Breast Cancer." *American Journal of Epidemiology*, vol. 139, no. 10, May 15, 1994, pp. 1001-1007.

———. "Estrogen Replacement Therapy and Risk of Fatal Colon Cancer in a Prospective Cohort of Postmenopausal Women." *Journal of the National Cancer Institute*, vol. 87, no. 7, April 5, 1995, pp. 517-523.

Cannistra, Stephen A., M.D. "Cancer of the Ovary." *New England Journal of Medicine*, vol. 329, no. 21, November 18, 1993, pp. 1550-1559.

Chang, Trina. "Expert Advice—Dr. Susan Love: Fighting Breast Cancer." *American Health*, June 1994.

Colditz, Graham A., M.B.B.S. Dr.P.H., Walter C. Willett, M.D., Andrea Rotnitzky, Ph.D., and JoAnn E. Manson, M.D. "Weight Gain as a Risk Factor for Clinical Diabetes Mellitus in Women." *Annals of Internal Medicine*, vol. 122, no. 7, April 1, 1995, pp. 481-486.

Collins, Francis S., M.D., Ph.D. "BRCA1—Lots of Mutations, Lots of Dilemmas." *New England Journal of Medicine*, vol. 334, no. 3, pp. 186-188.

Conkling, Winifred. "Pesticide Perspectives." *American Health*, October 1994.

Davis, Devra Lee, Ph.D., M.P.H., and Susan M. Love, M.D., "Mammographic Screening." *Journal of the American Medical Association*, vol. 271, no. 12, pp. 152-153.

DeCosse, Jerome J., M.D., George J. Tsioulias, M.D., and Judith S. Jacobson, M.P.H. "Colorectal Cancer: Detection, Treatment and Rehabilitation." CA—A Cancer Journal for Clinicians, vol. 44, no. 1, January/February 1994, pp. 27-42.

———. "Diet and Breast Cancer." Harvard Women's Health Watch, vol. 8, no. 11, April 1995, p. 1.

Dupont, William D., Ph.D., David L. Page, M.D., Fritz F. Parl, M.D., Ph.D., Cindy L. Vnenck-Jones, Ph.D., Walton D. Plummer, Jr., B.S., Margaret S. Rados, M.A., and Peggy A. Schuyler, R.N. "Long-Term Risk of Breast Cancer in Women with Fibroadenoma." New England Journal of Medicine, vol. 331, no. 1, July 7, 1994, pp. 10-15.

Eley, J. William, M.D., M.P.H., Holly A. Hill, M.D., Ph.D., Vivian W. Chen, Ph.D., Donald F. Austin, M.D., M.P.H., Margaret N. Wesley, Ph.D., Hyman B. Muss, M.D., Raymond S. Greenberg, M.D., Ph.D., Ralph J. Coates, Ph.D., Pelayo Correa, M.D., Carol K. Redmond, Sc.D., Carrie P. Hunger, M.D., Allen A. Herman, Ph.D., M.B.Ch.B., Robert Kurman, M.D., Robert Blacklow, M.D., Sam Shapiro, and Brenda K. Edwards, Ph.D. "Racial Differences in Survival from Breast Cancer." Journal of the American Medical Association, vol. 272, no. 12, September 28, 1994, pp. 947-954.

Ettinger, Bruce, M.D., and Deborah Grady, M.D. "The Waning Effect of Postmenopausal Estrogen Therapy on Osteoporosis." New England Journal of Medicine, vol. 329, no. 16, October 14, 1993, pp. 1192-1193.

Executive Committee for the Asymptomatic Carotid Atherosclerosis Study, "Endarterectomy for Asymptomatic Carotid Artery Stenosis." Journal of the American Medical Association, vol. 273, no. 18, May 10, 1995, pp. 1421-1428.

Falkeborn, Margareta, M.D., Ingemar Persson, Ph.D., Andras Terent, Ph.D., Hans-Olov Adami, Ph.D., Hans Lithell, Ph.D., and Reinhold Bergstrom, Ph.D. "Hormone Replacement Therapy and the Risk of Stroke." Archives of Internal Medicine, vol. 153, May 24, 1993, pp. 1201-1209.

Felson, David T., M.D., M.P.H., Yuquing Zhang, D.Sc., Marian T. Hannah, M.P.H., Douglas P. Kiel, M.D., M.P.H., Peter W. F. Wilson, M.D., and Jennifer Anderson, Ph.D. "The Effect of Postmenopausal Estrogen Therapy on Bone Density in Elderly Women." New England Journal of Medicine, vol. 329, no. 16, October 14, 1993, pp. 1141-46.

Fielding, Jonathan E., M.D., M.P.H. "Smoking and Women: Tragedy of the Majority." *New England Journal of Medicine*, vol. 317, no. 21, November 19, 1987, pp. 1343-1345.

Fletcher, Suzanne W., William Black, Russell Harris, Barbara K. Rimer, and Sam Shapiro. "Report of the International Workshop on Screening for Breast Cancer." *Journal of the National Cancer Institute*, vol. 85, no. 20, October 20, 1993, pp. 1644-1656.

Fontham, Elizabeth T.H., Dr.P.H., Pelayo Correa, M.D., Peggy Reynolds, Ph.D., Anna Wu-Williams, Ph.D., Patricia A. Buffler, Ph.D., Raymond S. Greenberg, M.D., Ph.D., Vivian W. Chen, Ph.D., Toni Alterman, Ph.D., Peggy Boyd, Ph.D., Donald F. Austin, M.D., Jonathan Liff, Ph.D., "Environmental Tobacco Smoke and Lung Cancer in Nonsmoking Women." *Journal of the American Medical Association*, vol. 271, no. 2, June 8, 1994, pp. 1752-1769.

Foster, Kenneth R., Linda S. Erdreich, and John E. Moulder, "Weak Electromagnetic Fields and Cancer in the Context of Risk Assessment." *Proceedings of the IEEE*, vol. 85, no. 5, May, 1997, pp. 733-746.

Freedman, Laurence S., Ross L. Prentice, Carolyn Clifford, William Harlan, Maureen Henderson, and Jacques Rossouw. "Dietary Fat and Breast Cancer: Where Are We?" *Journal of the National Cancer Institute*, vol. 85, no. 10, May 19, 1993, pp. 764-765.

Fuchs, Charles S., M.D., Edward L. Giovannucci, M.D., Graham A. Coltitz, M.B., B.S., David J. Hunter, M.B., B.S., Frank E. Spitzer, M.D., and Walter C. Willett, M.D. "A Prospective Study of Family History and the Risk of Colorectal Cancer." *New England Journal of Medicine*, vol. 331, no. 25, December 22, 1994, pp. 1669-1674.

Fuchs, Charles S., M.D., Meir J. Stampher, M.D., Graham A. Coltitz, M.B., B.S., Edward L. Giovannucci, M.D., JoAnn Manson, M.S., Irchiro Kawachi, M.B., Ch.B., David J. Hunter, M.B., B.S., Susan E. Hankinson, R.N., Sc.D., Charles H. Hennekens, M.D., Bernard Rosner, Ph.D., Frank E. Spitzer, M.D., and Walter C. Willett, M.D. "Alcohol Consumption and Mortality among Women." *New England Journal of Medicine*, vol. 332, no. 19, May 11, 1995, pp. 1246-1250.

Garg, Rekha, M.D., M.S., Diane K. Wagener, Ph.D., and Jennifer H. Madans, Ph.D. "Alcohol Consumption and Risk of Heart Disease in Women." *Archives of Internal Medicine*, vol. 153, May 24, 1993, pp. 1211-1216.

Gastrin, Gisela, M.D., Anthony B. Miller, M.B., F.R.C.P., Teresa To, Ph.D., Kristan J. Aronson, Ph.D., Claus Wall, M.Sc., Matti Hakama, Ph.D., Kristi Louhivuori, M.D., and Eero Pukkala, M.A. "Incidence and Mortality from Breast Cancer in the Mama Program for Breast Screening in Finland, 1974–1986." *Cancer*, vol. 73, no. 8, April 15, 1994, pp. 2168-2174.

Giovannucci, Edward, Graham A. Colditz, Meir J. Stampfer, David Hunter, Bernard A. Rosner, Walter C. Willett, and Frank E. Speizer. "A Prospective Study of Cigarette Smoking and Risk of Colorectal Adenoma and Colorectal Cancer in U.S. Women." *Journal of the National Cancer Institute*, vol. 86, no. 3, February 2, 1994, pp. 192-199.

Giovannucci, Edward, M.D., Sc.D., Eric B. Rimm, Sc.D., Meir J. Stampfer, M.D., Dr.P.H., Graham A. Colditz, M.D., Dr.P.H., Alberto Ascherio, M.D., M.P.H., Dr.P.H., and Walter C. Willett, M.D., Dr.P.H. "Aspirin Use and the Risk of Colorectal Cancer and Adenoma in Male Health Professionals." *Annals of Internal Medicine*, vol. 121, no. 4, August 15, 1994, pp. 241-246.

Giovannucci, G., M.B.B.Ch. (Wits) and V.U. Fritz, F.C.P. (SA), Ph.D. "Transient Ischemic Attacks in Younger and Older Patients: A Comparative Study of 798 Patients in South Africa." *Stroke*, vol. 24, no. 7, July 1993, pp. 947-953.

Greenberg, E. Robert, M.D., John A. Baron, M.D., Tor D. Tosteson, Sc.D., Daniel H. Freeman, Jr., Ph.D., Gerald J. Beck, Ph.D., John H. Bond, M.D., Thomas A. Colacchio, M.D., John A. Coller, M.D., Harold D. Frankl, M.D., Robert W. Haile, Dr.P.H., Jack S. Mandel, Ph.D., David W. Nierenberg, M.D., Richard Rothstein, M.D., Dale C. Snover, M.D., Marguerite M. Stevens, Ph.D., Robert W. Summers, M.D., and Rosalind U. van Stolk, M.D. "A Clinical Trial of Antioxidant Vitamins to Prevent Colorectal Adenoma." *New England Journal of Medicine*, vol. 331, no. 3, July 21, 1994, pp. 141-147.

————— ."Is It a Stroke?" *Consumer Reports Health Letter*, vol. 2, no. 6, June 1990, p. 45.

Grimes, David A., M.D. "Primary Prevention of Ovarian Cancer." *Journal of the American Medical Association*, vol. 270, no. 23, December 15, 1993, pp. 2855-2856.

Grodstein, Francine, Charles H. Hennekens, Graham A. Colditz, David J. Hunter, and Meir J. Stampfer. "A Prospective Study of Permanent Hair Dye Use and Hematopoietic Cancer." *Journal of the National Cancer Institute*, vol. 86, no. 19, October 5, 1994, pp. 1466-1470.

Gross, Thomas P., M.D., M.P.H., and James J. Schlesselman, Ph.D. "The Estimated Effect of Oral Contraceptive Use on the Cumulative Risk of Epithelial Ovarian Cancer." *Obstetrics & Gynecology*, vol. 83, no. 3, March 1994, pp. 421-424.

Hankinson, Susan E., Sc.D., David J. Hunter M.B., B.S., Graham A. Colditz, M.B., B.S., Walter C. Willett, M.D., Meir J. Stampfer, M.D., Bernard Rosner, Ph.D., Charles H. Hennekens, M.D., and Frank E. Speizer, M.D. "Tubal Ligation, Hysterectomy, and Risk of Ovarian Cancer: A Prospective Study." *Journal of the American Medical Association*, vol. 23, no. 270, December 15, 1993, pp. 2813-2818.

Harlow, Bernard L., and Noel S. Weiss. "Homocysteine—the Next Treatable Risk Factor?" *Harvard Heart Letter*, vol. 6, no. 11, July 1996, pp. 1-2.

Healy, Bernadine, M.D. "PEPI in Perspective: Good Answers Spawn Pressing Questions." *Journal of the American Medical Association*, vol. 273, no. 3, January 18, 1995, pp. 240-241.

Hershey, Linda A., M.D., Ph.D. "Gender Differences in Cerebrovascular Disease." *Neurology Chronicle*, vol. 3, no. 6, October 1993, pp. 1-4.

————. "Stroke Prevention in Women: Role of Aspirin versus Ticlopidine." *American Journal of Medicine*, vol. 91, September 1991, pp. 288-292.

Howe, Geoffrey R. "High-Fat Diet and Breast Cancer Risk: The Epidemiological Evidence." *Journal of the American Medical Association*, vol. 268, no. 15, October 21, 1992, pp. 2080-2081.

Hurt, Richard D., Lowell C. Dale, M.D., Paul A. Fredrickson, M.D., Casey C. Caldwell, M.D., Gary A. Lee, M.D., Richard P. Offord, M.S., Gary G. Lauger, M.S., Zrinka Marusic, M.D., Lewis W. Neese, M.D., and Thomas G. Lundberg, M.D., "Nicotine Patch Therapy for Smoking Cessation Combined with Physician Advice and Nurse Follow-up." *Journal of the American Medical Association*, vol. 271, no. 8, February 23, 1994, pp. 595-600.

Itri, Loretta, M.D., F.A.C.P. "Women and Lung Cancer." *Public Health Reports Supplement*, July-August 1986, pp. 92-96.

Jensen, Phyliss Marie, R.N., Ph.D., and Robert B. Coambs, Ph.D. "Health and Behavioral Predictors of Success in an Intensive Smoking Cessation Program for Women." *Women & Health*, vol. 21, no. 1, 1994, pp. 57-72.

Kaufman, Steven C., M.D., M.S., Robert Spirtas, Dr.P.H., F.A.C.E., and Nancy J. Alexander, Ph.D. "Do Fertility Drugs Cause Ovarian Tumors?" *Journal of Women's Health*, vol. 4, no. 3, June 1995, pp. 247-59.

Kawachi, Ichiro, M.B., Ch.B., Graham A. Colditz, M.D, Meir J. Stampfer, M.D., Walter C. Willett, M.D., JoAnn E. Manson, M.D., Frank E. Speizer, M.D., and Charles H. Hennekens, M.D. "Prospective Study of Shift Work and Risk of Coronary Heart Disease in Women." *Circulation*, vol. 92, no. 11, December 1, 1995, pp. 3178-3182.

Kawachi, Ichiro, M.B., Ch.B., Graham A. Colditz, M.D., Meir J. Stampfer, M.D., Walter C. Willett, M.D., JoAnn E. Manson, M.D., Bernard Rosner, Ph.D., Frank E. Speizer, M.D., and Charles H. Hennekens, M.D. "Smoking Cessation and Decreased Risk of Stroke in Women." *Journal of the American Medical Association*, vol. 269, no. 2, January 13, 1993, pp. 232-236.

Keller, Colleen, Ph.D., R.N., F.N.P., Julie Fleury, Ph.D., R.N., and Debra L. Bergstrom, M.S., R.N., C.C.R.N. "Risk Factors for Coronary Heart Disease in African-American Women." *Cardiovascular Nursing*, vol. 31, no. 2, March/April 1995, pp. 9-15.

Kelsey, Jennifer L., Editor, "Breast Cancer" (special edition). *Epidemiological Reviews*, vol. 15, no. 1, 1993.

Kelsey, Jennifer L., Ph.D., and Esther M. John, Ph.D. "Lactation and the Risk of Breast Cancer," *New England Journal of Medicine*, vol. 330, no. 2, January 13, 1994, 136-137.

Kelsey, Jennifer L., and Pamela H. Horn-Ross. "Breast Cancer: Magnitude of the Problem and Descriptive Epidemiology." *Epidemiology Review*, vol. 15, no. 1, 1993, pp. 7-16.

Kenford, Susan L., Michael C. Fiore, M.D., M.P.H., Douglas E. Jorenby, Ph.D., Stevens S. Smith, Ph.D., David Wetter, M.S., and Timothy B. Baker, Ph.D. "Predicting Smoking Cessation: Who Will Quit with and without the Nicotine Patch." *Journal of the American Medical Association*, vol. 271, no. 8, February 23, 1994, pp. 589-594.

Kerilikowske, Karla, M.D., Jeanette S. Brown, M.D., and Deborah G. Grady, M.D., M.P.H. "Should Women with Familial Ovarian Cancer Undergo Prophylactic Oophorectomy?" *Obstetrics & Gynecology*, vol. 80, no. 4, October 1992, pp. 700-707.

Kerlikowske, Karla, M.D., Deborah Grady, M.D., M.P.H., John Barclay, M.S., Edward A. Sickles, M.D., Abigail Eaton, M.P.H., and Virginia Ernster, Ph.D. "Positive Predictive Value of Screening Mammography by Age and Family History of Breast Cancer." *Journal of the American Medical Association*, vol. 270, no. 20, November 24, 1993, pp. 2444-2450.

Kern, Kenneth A., M.D., F.A.C.S. "Silicone Breast Implants: Carcinogenic Time Bomb or Toxic Tort Hoax." 12th Annual International Breast Cancer Conference, Miami Beach, Fla., March 16-18, 1995.

King, Abby C., Ph.D., William L. Haskell, Ph.D., Deborah R. Young, Ph.D., Roberta K. Oka, D.N.Sc., Marcia L. Stefanick, Ph.D. "Long-term Effects of Varying Intensities and Formats of Physical Activity on Participation Rates, Fitness and Lipoproteins in Men and Women Aged 50 to 65 Years." *Circulation*, vol. 19, no. 10, May 15, 1995, pp. 2596-2604.

Kliewer, Erich V., Ph.D., and Ken R. Smith. "Breast Cancer Mortality among Immigrants in Australia and Canada." *Journal of the National Cancer Institute*, vol. 87, no. 15, August 2, 1995, pp. 1154-1161.

Kokkinos, Peter F., Ph.D., John C. Holland, P.E.D., Andreas E. Pittaras, M.D., Puneet Narayan, M.D., Charles O. Dotson, Ph.D., and Vasilos Papademetriou, M.D., D.Sc., F.A.C.C. "Cardiorespiratory Fitness and Coronary Heart Disease Risk Factor Association in Women." *Journal of the American College of Cardiology*, vol. 26, no. 2, August 1995, pp. 358-364.

Krieger, Nancy, Mary S. Wolff, Robert A. Haitt, Marilyn Rivera, Joseph Vogelman, and Norman Orentreich. "Breast Cancer and Serum Organochlorines: A Prospective Study among White, Black and Asian Women." *Journal of the National Cancer Institute*, vol. 86, no. 8, April 20, 1994, pp. 589-599.

Kuller, Lewis, H., M.D., Dr.P.H. "A Time of Change: Early Signs of Atherosclerosis in Perimenopausal Women." Presented at the American Heart Association's 22nd Science Writers Forum, Santa Barbara, Calif., January 15-18, 1995.

Kushi, Lawrence H., Sc.D., Arron R. Folsom, M.D., Ronald J. Prineas,

M.B., B.S., Pamela J. Mink, M.P.H., Ying Wu, M.P.H., and Robert M. Bostick, M.D. "Dietary Antioxidant Vitamins and Death from Coronary Heart Disease in Postmenopausal Women." *New England Journal of Medicine*, vol. 334, no. 19, May 2, 1996, pp. 1156-1162.

Larsen, Natalie S. "Invasive Cervical Cancer Arising in Young White Females," *Journal of the National Cancer Institute*, vol. 86, no. 1, January 5, 1994, pp. 6-7.

Leitch, A. Marilyn, M.D., Gerald D. Dodd, M.D., Mary Cotsanza, M.D., Michael Linver, M.D., Peter Pressman, M.D., LaMar McGinnis, M.D., and Robert A. Smith, Ph.D. "American Cancer Society Guidelines for the Early Detection of Breast Cancer: Update 1997." *CA—A Cancer Journal for Clinicians*, vol. 47, no. 3, May/June 1997, pp. 150-153.

London, Stephanie J., Frank M. Sacks, Meir J. Stamper, I. Craig Henderson, Malcolm Maclure, Akiko Tomita, William C. Wood, Steven Remine, Nicholas J. Robert, Jan R. Dmochowski, and Walter C. Willett. "Fatty Acid Composition of the Subcutaneous Adipose Tissue and Risk of Proliferative Benign Breast Disease and Breast Cancer." *Journal of the National Cancer Institute*, vol. 85, no. 10, May 19, 1993, pp. 785-793.

Longnecker, Matthew P., Polly A. Newcomb, Robert Mittendorf, E. Robert Greenberg, Richard W. Clapp, Gregory F. Bogdan, John Baron, Brian MacMahon, and Walter C. Willett. "Risk of Breast Cancer in Relation to Lifetime Alcohol Consumption." *Journal of the National Cancer Institute*, vol. 87, no. 12, June 21, 1995, pp. 923-928.

Loomis, Dana P., Ph.D., David A. Savitz, and Cande V. Anath. "Breast Cancer Mortality Among Female Electrical Workers in the United States." *Journal of the National Cancer Institute*, vol. 86, no. 12, June 15, 1994, pp. 921-925.

Love, Betsy B., M.D., Maleah Grover-McKay, M.D., José Biller, M.D., Karim Rezai, M.D., and Charles R. McKay, M.D. "Coronary Artery Disease and Cardiac Events with Asymptomatic and Symptomatic Cerebrovascular Disease." *Stroke*, vol. 23, no. 7, July 1992, pp. 939-945.

Marenberg, Marjorie E., Ph.D., Neil Risch, Ph.D., Lisa F. Berkman, Ph.D., Birgitta Floderus, Ph.D., and Ulf De Faire, M.D., Ph.D.

"Genetic Susceptibility to Death from Coronary Heart Disease in a Study of Twins." *New England Journal of Medicine*, vol. 330, no. 15, pp. 1041-1046.

Miller, Anthony B., M.B., F.R.C.P. Cornelia J. Baines, M.D., M.Sc., Teresa To, Ph.D., Claus Wall, M.Sc. "Canadian National Breast Screening Study: Breast Cancer Detection and Death Rates among Women Aged 40 to 49 Years." *Canadian Medical Association Journal*, vol. 121, no. 4, pp. 1459-1488.

Morrison, Howard I., Ph.D., Douglas Schaubel, Marie Desmeules, M.Sc., and Donald T. Wigle, M.D., Ph.D. "Serum Folate and Risk of Fatal Coronary Heart Disease." *Journal of the American Medical Association*, vol. 275, no. 24, pp. 1893-1896.

Ness, Roberta B., M.D., M.P.H., Tamara Harris, M.D., M.S., Janet Cobb, M.P.H., Katherine M. Flegal, Ph.D., Jennifer L. Kelsey, Ph.D., Albert Balanger, M.D., Albert J. Stunkard, M.D., and Ralph B. D'Agostino, Ph.D. "Number of Pregnancies and the Subsequent Risk of Cardiovascular Disease." *New England Journal of Medicine*, vol. 328, no. 21, pp. 1529-1533.

Newcomb, Polly A., Ph.D., and Barry E. Storer, Ph.D. "Postmenopausal Use and Risk of Large-Bowel Cancer." *Journal of the National Cancer Institute*, vol. 87, no. 14, July 19, 1995, pp. 1067-1071.

Newcomb, Polly A., Ph.D., Barry E. Storer, Ph.D., Matthew P. Longnecker, M.D., Robert Mittendorf, M.D., E. Robert Greenberg, M.D., Richard W. Clapp, Sc.D., Kenneth P. Burke, M.D., Walter C. Willett, M.D., and Brian C. MacMahon, M.D. "Lactation and a Reduced Risk of Premenopausal Breast Cancer." *New England Journal of Medicine*, vol. 330, no. 2, January 13, 1994, pp. 81-87.

Paganini-Hill, Annlia, Ronald K. Ross, and Brian E. Henderson. "Postmenopausal Estrogen Treatment and Stroke: A Prospective Study." *British Medical Journal*, August 20-27, 1988, vol. 297, pp. 519-22.

Pashkow, Fredric J., M.D. "The Mona Lisa Smiles: Impact of Risk Factors for Coronary Artery Disease in Women." *Cleveland Clinic Journal of Medicine*, vol. 60, no. 5, September/October 1993.

Pate, Russell R., Ph.D., Michael Pratt, M.D., M.P.H., Steven N. Blair, P.E.D., William L. Haskell, Ph.D., Caroline A. Macera, Ph.D., Claude Bouchard, Ph.D., David Buchner, M.D., M.P.H., Walter Ettinger, M.D., Gregory W. Heath, D.H.Sc., Abby C. King, Ph.D.,

Andea Kriska, Ph.D., Arthur S. Leon, M.D., Bess H. Marcus, Ph.D., Jeremy Morris, M.D., Ralph S. Paffenbarger, Jr., M.D., Kevin Patrick, M.D., Michael L. Pollock, Ph.D., James M. Rippe, M.D., James Sallis, Ph.D., and Jack H. Wilmore, Ph.D. "Physical Activity and Public Health: A Recommendation from the Centers for Disease Control and Prevention and the American College of Sports Medicine." *Journal of the American Medical Association*, vol. 273, no. 5, February 1, 1995, pp. 402-407.

Piver, Steven M., M.D., and Ronald E. Hempling, M.D. "Screening for Gynecologic Malignancies in Primary Care: Ovarian Cancer." *Emergency Medicine*, March 1993, pp. 141-148.

Podolsky, Doug. "New Weapons That Might Defeat Stroke." *U.S. News & World Report*, April 13, 1992, pp. 66-73.

Pollack, Michael, Ph.D., and William R. Brechue, Ph.D. "Exercise Guidelines for the Older Woman." *Women's Health Digest*, vol. 1, no. 1, Winter 1995, pp. 31-33.

Recio, Fernando O, M.D. "Prophylactic Ooophorectomy with or without Hysterectomy." *Ovarian Plus International*, vol. 3, no. 2, Spring 1997, pp. 1-2.

Reichman, Marcia E., Joseph T. Judd, Christopher Longcope, Arthur Schatzin, Beverly A. Clevidence, Padmanabhan P. Nair, William S. Campbell, and Philip R. Taylor. "Effects of Alcohol Consumption on Plasma and Urinary Hormone Concentrations in Premenopausal Women." *Journal of the National Cancer Institute*, vol. 85, no. 9, May 5, 1993, pp. 722-726.

Rennie, Susan. "Breast Cancer Prevention: Diet vs. Drugs." *Ms.*, May/June 1993, pp. 38-46.

Rigel, Darrell S., M.D. "Malignant Melanoma: Perspectives on Incidence and Its Effects on Awareness, Diagnosis and Treatment." *CA—A Journal for Cancer Clinicians*, vol. 46, no. 4, July/August 1996, pp. 195-198.

Risch, Harvey A., Geoffrey R. Howe, Meera Jain, J. David Burch, Eric J. Holowaty, and Anthony B. Miller. "Are Female Smokers at Higher Risk for Lung Cancer Than Male Smokers?" *American Journal of Epidemiology*, vol. 138, no. 5, September 1, 1993, pp. 281-293.

Risch, Harvey A., Meera Jain, Lorraine D. Marrett, and Geoffrey R. Howe. "Dietary Fat Intake and Risk of Epithelial Ovarian Cancer."

Journal of the National Cancer Institute, vol. 86, no. 18, September 21, 1994, pp. 1409-1415.

Rodriquez, Carmen, Eugenia E. Calle, Ralph J. Coates, Heidi L. Miracle-McMahill, Michael J. Thun, and Clark W. Heath, Jr. "Estrogen Replacement Therapy and Fatal Ovarian Cancer," *American Journal of Epidemiology*, vol. 141, no. 9, September 1995, pp. 828-835.

Rookus, Matti A., and Flora E van Leeuwen. "Oral Contraceptives and Risk of Breast Cancer in Women Aged 20-54 Years." *The Lancet*, vol. 344, September 24, 1994, pp. 844-851.

Rosenthal, Dorothy L. "Automation and the Endangered Future of the Pap Test." *Journal of the National Cancer Institute*, vol. 90, no. 10, May 20, 1998, pp. 738-49.

Rossing, Mary Anne, D.V.M., Ph.D., Janet R. Daling, Ph.D., Noel S. Weiss, M.D., Dr. P.H., Donald E. Moore, M.D., and Steven G. Self, Ph.D. "Ovarian Cancer in a Cohort of Infertile Women." *New England Journal of Medicine*, vol. 31, no. 12, pp. 771-796.

Sandberg, Avery A., M.D., D.Sc. "Cancer Cytogenics for Clinicians." *CA—A Cancer Journal for Clinicians*, vol. 44, no. 3, May-June 1994, pp. 136-159.

Sharp, David. "The Quitter's Exercise Plan." *Health*, May/June 1994, pp. 69-76.

Shingleton, Hugh M., M.D., Roman L. Patrick, M.D., William W. Johnston, M.D., and Robert A. Smith, Ph.D. "The Current Status of the Papanicolaou Smear." *CA—A Cancer Journal for Clinicians*, vol. 45, no. 5, September/October 1995, pp. 305-320.

Shinton, Roger, and Gian Sigar. "Lifetime Exercise and Stroke." *British Medical Journal*, vol. 307, July 24, 1993, pp. 229-232.

Sickles, Edward A., M.D., and Daniel B. Kopans, M.D. "Mammographic Screening for Women Aged 40 to 49 Years: The Primary Care Practitioner's Dilemma." *Annals of Internal Medicine*, vol. 122, no. 7, April 1, 1995, pp. 534-537.

Silverstein, Melvin J., M.D., "Breast Cancer Diagnosis and Treatment after Augmentation Mammoplasty." 12th Annual International Breast Cancer Conference, Miami Beach, Fla., March 16-18, 1995.

Simon, Harvey B., M.D. "Can You Run Away from Cancer?" *Harvard Health Letter*, March 1992, pp. 5-7.

Smigel, Kara. "Aspirin's Next Conquest: Does It Prevent Colon Cancer?" *Journal of the National Cancer Institute*, vol. 86, no. 3, February 2, 1994, pp. 166-168.

———. "Group Defines Directions for Colorectal Cancer Screening." *Journal of the National Cancer Institute*, vol. 86, no. 13, July 6, 1994, pp. 958-960.

Sowers, James, M.D. "Modest Weight Gain and the Development of Diabetes: Another Perspective," *Annals of Internal Medicine*, vol. 122, no. 7, April 1, 1995, pp. 548-549.

Sox, Harold C., M.D. "Screening Mammography in Women Younger Than 50 Years of Age." Annals of Internal Medicine, vol. 122, no. 7, April 1, 1995, pp. 550-552.

Stampher, Meir J., M.D., Charles H. Hennekens, M.D., JoAnn E. Manson, M.D., Graham A. Colditz, M.B., B.S., Bernard Rosner, Ph.D., and Walter C. Willett, M.D., "Vitamin E Consumption and the Risk of Coronary Artery Disease in Women," *New England Journal of Medicine*, vol. 328, no. 20, May 20, 1993, pp. 1444-1449.

Steinberg, Daniel, M.D., Ph.D. "Antioxidant Vitamins and Coronary Heart Disease." *New England Journal of Medicine*, vol. 328, no. 20, May 20, 1993, pp. 1487-1488.

Talbott, Evelyn, David Guzick, Annette Clerici, Sarah Berga, Katherine Detre, Karl Weimer, and Lewis Kuller. "Coronary Heart Disease Risk Factors in Women with Polycystic Ovary Syndrome." *Arteriosclerosis, Thrombosis, and Vascular Biology*, vol. 15, no. 7, July 1995, pp. 821-825.

Tanne, Janice Hopkins. "Everything You Need to Know about Breast Cancer . . . but Were Afraid to Ask." *New York*, October 11, 1993, pp. 53-62.

Tarkan, Laurie. "The New 'Light' Physicals: Are They Healthy?" *Good Housekeeping*, June 1995, pp. 157-158.

Taylor, Pamela A., M.D., and Ann Ward, Ph.D. "Women, High-Density Lipoprotein Cholesterol, and Exercise." *Archives of Internal Medicine*, vol. 153, May 24, 1993, pp. 1178-1183.

Teneriello, Michael G., M.D., and Robert C. Park, M.D. "Early Detective of Ovarian Cancer." *CA—A Cancer Journal for Clinicians*, vol. 45, no. 2, March/April 1994, pp. 71-87.

The Writing Group for the PEPI Trial. "Effects of Estrogen or Estrogen/Progestin Regimens on Heart Disease Risk Factors in Postmenopausal Women." *Journal of the American Medical Association*, vol. 273, no. 3, January 18, 1995, pp. 199-208.

Thompson, Marilyn E., Roy A. Jensen, Patrice S. Obermiller, David L. Page, and Jeffrey T. Holt. "Decreased Espression of BRAC1 Accelerates Growth and Is Often Present during Sporadic Breast Cancer Progression." *Nature Genetics*, vol. 9, April 1995, pp. 444-450.

Thun, Michael J., M.D., M.S., Cathy A. Day-Lally, Eugenia E. Calle, Ph.D., W. Dana Flanders, M.D., D.Ph., and Clark W. Heath, Jr., M.D. "Excess Mortality among Cigarette Smokers: Changes in a 20-Year Interval." *American Journal of Public Health*, vol. 85, no. 9, September 1995, pp. 1223-1230.

Thun, Michael J., M.D., Mohan M. Namboodiri, B.S., and Clark W. Heath, Jr., M.D. "Aspirin Use and Reduced Risk of Fatal Colon Cancer." *New England Journal of Medicine*, vol. 325, no. 23, December 5, 1991, pp. 1593-1596.

Thun, Michael J., M.D., Sean F. Altekruse, Mohan M. Namboodiri, Eugenia E. Calle, Dena G. Myers and Clark W. Heath, Jr. "Hair Dye Use and Risk of Fatal Cancers in U.S. Women." *Journal of the National Cancer Institute*, vol. 86, no. 3, February 2, 1994, pp. 210-215.

Troisi, Rebecca J., Frank E. Speizer, Walter C. Willett, Dimitrios Trichopoulos, and Bernard Rosner. "Menopause, Postmenopausal Estrogen Preparations, and the Risk of Adult-Onset Asthma." *American Journal of Respiratory Critical Care Medicine*, vol. 162, no. 4, October 1995, pp. 1183-1188.

Weiss, Rick. "Estrogen in the Environment." *Washington Post Health*, January 25, 1994, pp. 10-14.

White, Emily, Kathleen E. Malone, Noel S. Weiss, and Janet R. Daling. "Breast Cancer among Young U.S. Women in Relation to Oral Contraceptive Use." *Journal of the National Cancer Institute*, vol. 86, no. 7, April 6, 1994, pp. 505-514.

Whittemore, Alice S. "The Risk of Ovarian Cancer after Treatment for Infertility." *New England Journal of Medicine*, vol. 31, no. 12, pp. 805-806.

Whittemore, Alice S., and Brian E. Henderson. "Dietary Fat and Breast Cancer: Where Are We?" *Journal of the National Cancer Institute*, vol. 85, no. 10, May 19, 1993, pp. 762-763.

Whittemore, Alice S., Robin Harris, Jacqueline Itnyr, and the Collaborative Ovarian Cancer Group. "Characteristics Relating to Ovarian Cancer Risk: Collaborative Analysis of 12 U.S. Case-Control Studies: Part II, Invasive Epithelial Ovarian Cancers in White Women." *American Journal of Epidemiology*, vol. 136, no. 10, November 15, 1992, pp. 1184-1203.

Willett, Walter C., M.D., David J. Hunter, M.B., B.S., Meir J. Stampfer, M.D., Graham Colditz, M.D., B.S., JoAnn E. Manson, M.D., Donna Spiegelman, D.Sc., Bernard Rosner, Ph.D., Charles H. Hennekens, M.D., and Frank E. Speizer, M.D., "Dietary Fat and Fiber in Relation to Risk of Breast Cancer." *Journal of the American Medical Association*, vol. 268, no. 15, October 21, 1992, pp. 2037-2044.

Willett, Walter C., M.D., Meir J. Stampfer, M.D., Graham Colditz, M.D., Bernard Rosner, Ph.D., and Frank E. Speizer, M.D. "Relation of Meat, Fat, and Fiber Intake to the Risk of Colon Cancer in a Prospective Study among Women." *New England Journal of Medicine*, vol. 323, no. 24, December 13, 1990, pp. 1664-1672.

Wolff, Mary S., Paolo, G. Toniolo, Eric W. Lee, Marilyn Rivera, and Neil Dubin. "Blood Levels of Organochlorine Residues and Risk of Breast Cancer." *Journal of the National Cancer Institute*, vol. 85, no. 8, April 21, 1993, pp. 648-652.

Wong-Ho Chow, Gloria Gridley, Olo Nyrén, Martha S. Linet, Anders Ekbom, Joseph F. Fraumeni, Jr., and Hans-Olov Adami. "Risk of Pancreatic Cancer Following Diabetes Mellitus: A Nationwide Cohort Study in Sweden." *Journal of the National Cancer Institute*, vol. 87, no. 12, June 21, 1995, pp. 930-931.

Zang, Edith A., and Ernst L. Wynder. "Differences in Lung Cancer Risk between Men and Women: Examination of the Evidence." *Journal of the National Cancer Institute*, vol. 88, no. 3/4, February 21, 1996, pp. 183-192.

INDEX